From Luke to Liz, from Chloe to Justin, the people in this book could be anyone you know—including you. Because you like them and identify with them, you begin to believe, for real, that you, too, might get an STD and suffer the consequences. Every young person who is having sex or thinking about having sex should read this book.

—Diane F. Clark, RN, Family Life Educator, Chesterfield County, Virginia

What do teenagers, soccer moms, CEOs, and medical students have in common? Each is at risk of contracting an STD. *Seductive Delusions* illustrates the stories behind sexually transmitted disease statistics, giving faces and emotions to these contagious infections. Don't be surprised if you find yourself thinking, "That sounds like me!" Dr. Grimes gives us the much-needed reality check and the necessary information to prevent us from becoming a character in *Seductive Delusions*.

—Ashley Wietsma, writer of the *Johns Hopkins Newsletter* column "Orgasmic Chemistry"

Students reported that the stories of people like them made sexually transmitted diseases seem more real and the stories stuck with them much better than hearing just facts and stats.

—Patty Amidon, Coordinator of Health and Peer Education, Alfred State College

Enthralls us with gripping tales of real people facing illness and tragedy. And the kick comes with how Grimes wisely brings the reader to be motivated to avoid the infectious danger that is truly out there. (I'm getting copies for my kids.) . . . Should be a required textbook for all high school health classes.

—Richard P. Holm, MD, National Association of Medical Communicators

One of my students said, "Is it weird if some of the people in my group are reading this book like it is *The Hunger Games*?" I thought that was a compliment to Dr. Grimes and *Seductive Delusions*!

—Schoolteacher

Dr. Jill Grimes has found an innovative way to connect with young people. By telling the stories of everyday people, she speaks to a sizeable population who assumes that because they don't fall into a traditionally defined "risk" group, they are not at risk for STDs.

—Ellen Friedrichs, sexedvice.com

All of the students really get into the book (you can hear a pin drop in class) and seem to connect to the book.

—Schoolteacher

The book is a good gift for the teen in your life who just might be contemplating getting into a relationship (sexual or not).

—Sacramento Book Review

Anyone who is sexually active is at risk of contracting an STD. By sharing these very real experiences, Dr. Grimes shows how everyday people can contract one of these preventable diseases. Everyone, including physicians, can learn from the stories in this book.

—Robert E. Rakel, MD, Baylor College of Medicine

This is [a book] we wholeheartedly recommend for adolescents, their parents, and teachers.

—Parenting Press

Grimes debunks the "seductive delusion" that people cannot catch STDs if they choose the "right" partner.

—*Library Journal*

Read the book from cover to cover. . . . Knowledge is power.

—**Healthbolt.net**

I would highly recommend this book to all sexually active young people. It is eye-opening and disturbing in the right sort of way.

—**www.getbetterhealth.com**

Highly recommended.

—**Linda Carlson, PEP Talk**

seduct*ive delusions

seductive*

delusions

HOW EVERYDAY PEOPLE CATCH STIs

[*second edition*]

JILL GRIMES, MD

Johns Hopkins University Press
Baltimore

Note to the Reader: This book is not meant to substitute for medical care of people with sexually transmitted infections, and treatment should not be based solely on its contents. Instead, treatment must be developed in a dialogue between the individual and his or her physician. Our book has been written to help with that dialogue.

This book presents accounts of people who have an STI. None of the characters portrayed here are actual people; any resemblance to actual people is purely coincidental.

Drug dosage: The author and publisher have made reasonable efforts to determine that the selection of drugs discussed in this text conform to the practices of the general medical community. The medications described do not necessarily have specific approval by the US Food and Drug Administration for use in the diseases for which they are recommended. In view of ongoing research, changes in governmental regulation, and the constant flow of information relating to drug therapy and drug reactions, the reader is urged to check the package insert of each drug for any change in indications and dosage and for warnings and precautions. This is particularly important when the recommended agent is a new and/or infrequently used drug.

Printed in the United States of America on acid-free paper
9 8 7 6 5 4 3 2 1

The 2008 edition was published as *Seductive Delusions: How Everyday People Catch STDs.*

Johns Hopkins University Press
2715 North Charles Street
Baltimore, Maryland 21218-4363
www.press.jhu.edu

Library of Congress cataloging-in-publication data will be found at the end of this book.

A catalog record for this book is available from the British Library.

Special discounts are available for bulk purchases of this book. For more information, please contact Special Sales at 410-516-6936 or specialsales@press.jhu.edu.

Johns Hopkins University Press uses environmentally friendly book materials, including recycled text paper that is composed of at least 30 percent post-consumer waste, whenever possible.

To all my patients,

in thanks for your trust

Contents

Preface

THE EVERYDAY WORLD OF medicine has raced forward in the years since the first edition of this book was published. Electronic medical records have all but replaced paper charts, and communication with patients often takes place by voice mail or texting over smartphones and tablets, rather than via landline phones and paper handouts. Guidelines for cervical cancer prevention and Pap tests have changed dramatically, and HPV vaccines are now routinely recommended for all children (boys and girls). Sexually transmitted diseases (STDs) are now referred to as sexually transmitted infections (STIs), primarily because the word "disease" implies a specific, easily identifiable set of symptoms, and most of these infections are largely silent. What has not changed in the past few years is the seductive delusion that if we choose the "right" people, there won't be any adverse emotional or physical consequences from sexual activity. No one seems to believe that STIs occur within *their* peer group.

In the exam room, patients who are diagnosed with a sexually transmitted infection invariably look at us in shock and dismay, sincerely wondering how this could possibly have happened to them.

When our patients are students, their concerned parents are often angry, confused, or bitter, blaming themselves or broadly accusing "society." The media certainly portray STIs as a distant issue, affecting only the social outcasts of our society. Although we hear about new hookups between superstars every week, when was the last time we heard of an actor or supermodel catching an STI? The common belief is that STIs belong with prostitutes and promiscuous people and not with "people like us." Although people who have sex with multiple partners do have higher risks, the population most primary care physicians treat for STIs is not whom you might expect. What I want to make clear is that *we discover STIs in everyone*, including cheerleaders, valedictorians, athletes, and professionals of all disciplines. No social class, economic class, culture, religion, gender, or race is immune.

Included here are the condensed stories of people who are just like you and me—and who get an STI. My hope is that sharing the stories of successful, intelligent, attractive women and men as they are stunned with the diagnosis of a sexually transmitted infection will help you remember the facts of STI prevention as easily as you remember the details of a television series. As you read and live through each situation—seeing, feeling, and experiencing the action through the characters—I hope that the details of transmission, diagnosis, and treatment become a firm memory for you, rather than facts to memorize. Instead of an emergency appendectomy with Dr. McDreamy on *Grey's Anatomy*, here we join Logan in an urgent care clinic in Florida, spending his last day of spring break receiving a shot of antibiotics for a newly acquired STI, and we get to know Ashley, an unsuspecting college student who realizes she was a victim of sexual assault while under the influence of a date-rape drug.

This book is for everyone, because everyone needs to know how STIs are spread, how to avoid getting one, what the symptoms are, and how they are diagnosed and treated. Because this book presents accurate information on STIs through the stories of characters who get these infections as actual people do, I hope you will find it readable and interesting—an example of how crucial information can be conveyed without being didactic or boring. I was happy to learn that when high school teachers in Texas assigned the earlier edition of this book to their students, the response was overwhelmingly positive. Teachers consistently reported, "Once they opened the book and started the reading assignment, you could hear a pin drop—and that never happens in my classroom." Feedback from students has been rewarding, with this being perhaps my favorite compliment: "Is it weird if . . . the people in my group are reading this book like it is *The Hunger Games*?" I am gratified that these stories have opened up important conversations not only in classrooms but also in homes.

Health education is an area where knowledge can prevent heartache and misery and save lives, but only if the information is read, digested, and retained. This book helps people in and out of the classroom take on this important information and absorb it. In the earlier edition, I thought I would try a different approach from that taken in standard sex education materials, and the results were so positive that an updated edition is now needed. Stories are far more powerful than statistics, and they are far easier to share and discuss. I provide accurate medical information while clearly (yet not graphically) illustrating how STIs are spread through other types of sexual intimacy beyond intercourse. The ultimate goal, of course, is to help you to avoid acquiring an STI, which you may have for the rest of your life.

As you begin this book, please keep in mind that you can read all of these stories in the order I've presented them, or you can start with any specific STI, whether you are worried that you might already have this STI or that you may get it or give it to someone else. (If you do have such concerns, the best thing you can do is see your physician for testing and advice before you engage in any additional sexual activity.) The story of most of the STIs is told through the perspective of one male and one female character, to allow you to identify with your own gender and to gain some understanding of and empathy with what a partner might be experiencing. After each pair of stories, a fact sheet provides a quick reference for the symptoms, treatment, prevention, and other important information about that STI, as well as answers to frequently asked questions. Each section concludes with some resources for additional information.

Your sexual health today has implications that range far into the future. Decisions made early in your life regarding sexual activity can impact your future fertility, self-worth, and even choice of a life partner. No one intends to catch any disease, and *you can't go back and make a different decision* once you've contracted a viral STI or developed scarring in your reproductive organs.

In an attempt to respect our patients' choices, we doctors may not do enough to describe the potential emotional hazards of sexual encounters. The decision to be sexually intimate should involve much more than the knowledge of how to prevent pregnancy and how to avoid STIs. Healthy relationships thrive on open communication, mutual respect, and trust. These qualities should apply universally, including to discussions and decisions about physical intimacy. Understanding the emotional and physical consequences of sexual activity helps empower people to talk meaningfully and honestly with a prospective partner before impulsively reacting to their hormones, perceived expectations, passion, or even true love.

I wrote this book because I worry about every patient who has agonized in my office when I told them that they have a sexually transmitted infection. Unfortunately, I have seen hundreds of patients with STIs for each character portrayed in this book. (Any resemblance of a character in the book to any specific patient is thus purely coincidental.) Most of the medical issues described here apply to STIs acquired through both homosexual and heterosexual intimacy. I have not included stories specifically about gay men or lesbians or bisexual or transgender people, however, because I could not find a reasonable way to make the book representative without making it twice as long. Specific information for homosexual partners is included in the fact sheets and FAQ sections.

Pregnancy also is not addressed in this book, although it is clearly another potential consequence of unplanned or unprotected sex. While an unplanned pregnancy can bring joy, it also can cause anguish. However, in this book, I focus on how people catch sexually transmitted infections.

After reading the fact sheets on each STI, readers may question the effectiveness of condoms in preventing infection. Condoms have been proven to work best for decreasing the transmission of STIs carried through semen—HIV, chlamydia, gonorrhea, and trichomoniasis. They do not offer the same level of protection against diseases transmitted through direct contact, such as herpes, HPV, syphilis, and pubic lice. To be maximally effective, condoms must be used consistently, correctly, and for all types of genital contact, including oral-genital. Breakage, slippage, inconsistent and improper use (such as putting on the condom after pre-ejaculate has appeared) lead to condom failure rates of nearly twenty percent.

I learned long ago not to judge people, and I hope this book reflects my intent to create a nonmoralistic approach to the problem of STIs. This is not a book that says you're bad if you have sex. It is a practical, informative book that says look, here are the facts about what you risk medically if you have sex. I hope that you learn and benefit from the experiences depicted here and use the information to protect yourself, your friends, and your loved ones.

Many wonderful people deserve thanks. First is my dear friend Frank Domino, MD, for his enthusiastic support from the very first story, before there was a book, to confirming the medical accuracy at the end.

Friends and colleagues have been a constant support, provided encouragement, and prompted me to continue whenever I stalled. Special thanks to Adam, Elise, Lynn, and Rich Lampert for your friendship, suggestions, and never-ending promotion of this book. Huge appreciation also goes to Lorna, Coni, Brenda, Rhonda, Liza, Daniela, Barbara, and Mary for listening to my ideas, giving me valuable feedback, making me laugh, and providing the zeal to continue. Other "mommydocs" cheered every step of the way, especially my close friends Dr. Kristyn Fagerberg, Dr. Susan Kent, and Dr. Julia Sargent.

I thank all my wonderful patients for trusting me with the care of their health, especially those families I have had the privilege of knowing and treating for many years. I miss my Westlake Family Practice family, but adore my urgent care family at the University of Texas's Health Services.

I now understand why authors thank their editors. Huge thanks to Jacqueline Wehmueller for always staying positive, listening to my concerns, expertly streamlining stories, and recognizing a need for an updated second edition. My copyeditor, Merryl Sloane, beautifully polished the flow of dialogue and meticulously confirmed details in this edition; many thanks for your hard work.

To my parents, who continue their guidance from above, "Saint Janet" and Dad, "ye ole professor," thanks for instilling my love of books, a desire to teach, and the drive to complete this project because "anything worth doing is worth doing right." To our newest angel, Bene-Mimi, my sweet RN mother-in-law, much love; we miss you terribly. To my sister, Linda, thanks for sharing your expertise as a gynecologist. To John and the rest of our family, love and thanks. To our wonderful daughters, Brittany and Nicole, a million thanks for cheering me on—despite the awkward topic. This project started long before they were old enough to understand the content, and I offer huge kudos to our now-teenage girls who have graciously survived their mom being an STI expert and frequently speaking on the topic to their peers, to their organizations, or, even worse, on the radio. Somehow it was never my *Doctor Radio* interviews on influenza or diabetes that aired when the girls were carpooling to and from dance class . . . only the STI segments! Finally, to my incredible husband, Drew, what can I say? You are amazing and always have given me your unconditional support, love, and laughter, even when my career took an unexpected detour through a universally uncomfortable subject. These first two decades of marriage have flown by, and I cannot wait to see what the next ones bring. Love you!

seduct*ive delusions

HERPES SIMPLEX VIRUS

1: Grace

"THE DOCTOR WILL BE in to see you shortly," the perky medical assistant at the university health center had chirped. But that was nearly twenty minutes ago. Long enough for Grace to flip through all of the dated *People* magazines, memorize the stop smoking poster, and count the tiles in the floor. It was also long enough for the sweat on the back of her thighs to soak the paper on the exam table, causing it to stick to her and rip as she shifted nervously. Grace fretfully twirled a strand of her straight, shoulder-length blonde hair. She was freezing in the paper-thin gown, yet anxiety was making her perspire. How could she have ended up in this spot? As a medical student, she felt as though she belonged on the other side of the exam table.

Her thoughts drifted back to that first day in class. The professor was finishing up his introduction to the trials and tribulations of medical school, and he had one final admonition. "Despite popular belief, med school is not all the romantic fun and games that you see on TV shows like *Grey's Anatomy*. I would strongly suggest that you choose not to hook up with your classmates. You will have to work side by side with these people for the next four years—sleep deprived, mentally and physically exhausted. Believe me, you don't need the extra emotional baggage that relationships will bring." Everyone had shared a laugh, but within a month, almost half of the class was romantically involved, and Grace was no exception.

In the gross anatomy lab, four students were assigned to each cadaver. Grace was paired up with Miguel on the right side of the body, and two other classmates had the left side. Miguel's sense of humor attracted Grace, although he was not her usual physical type. Both of Grace's former college boyfriends had been very tall, thin, and wiry. In contrast, Miguel was only around five foot nine, about three inches taller than Grace, with an extremely muscular build that reflected his frequent competition in triathlons. Grace and Miguel had immediate chemistry. Their rush of nervous adrenaline from that first day of actually dissecting a human body had carried them into a quickly deepening relationship—first as study partners, then as partners between the sheets. Grace had been shocked by how fast they had ended up sleeping together. She was not a virgin, but had only had sex with two other men in her life, her long-term college boyfriends. Perhaps it was the excitement of her life plans coming together. She had always dreamed of becoming a doctor, and now here she was in her first year of medical school. Grace was bursting with confidence and enthusiasm. Miguel felt exactly the same way, and a celebratory hug and kiss at the end of their first round of practice exams had sparked their passion. Now, they had been together almost six months.

Last month, just after her period, Grace had developed an incredibly painful spot in her crotch. She had been certain that it was a pressure sore from her new jeans. Grace had bought them because she loved the decorative stitching down the sides, but she had hoped they would stretch out a bit, since they were a little too snug. As she sat through the marathon classroom and online lectures, followed by many more hours in the library or at Miguel's condo studying for their exams, a seam in the jeans must have rubbed a tender spot. However, when the sore area began to ache and burn again after her period this month, Grace was afraid that the discomfort had nothing to do with her jeans. So here she sat at the gynecologist's office, dreading the upcoming exam. The doorknob rattled, and Grace's knuckles whitened as her grip on the exam table involuntarily clamped down.

"Hi. I'm Dr. Chen. So what seems to be the problem today?," said the doctor as she walked in. Grace couldn't believe how young her doctor looked. Grace felt like Dr. Chen should be one of her classmates, rather than her doctor, but overall she just was relieved that the doctor was female. Seeing a male doctor for this type of exam would have been even more embarrassing.

Grace took a deep breath to compose herself, wanting to appear cool and intelligent. "Well, I appear to have a recurring painful red sore. I noticed it for the first time last month, right after my period. The blisters lasted around a week or so, and I thought they were from wearing some new jeans. Unfortunately, they came back this month in the same spot, and now I'm worried that it might be . . ."

"Herpes?," filled in Dr. Chen.

Grace burst into tears. How humiliating. She could barely choke out a reply. "Yes, of course, that's what I'm afraid that it is."

Dr. Chen handed her a tissue and smiled reassuringly. "Let me ask you a few questions, and then we'll take a look."

Grace sniffed and nodded her head in reply.

"Okay," said Dr. Chen. "Have you ever had a sexually transmitted infection before?"

A fresh wave of tears washed over Grace. "No. I've only had two previous partners, and I never even had a yeast infection."

Dr. Chen smiled. "Sorry. I know these are very personal questions," she said, "but it's important that I get your past history before I examine you. What kind of birth control are you using?"

"I'm on the pill," Grace replied.

"Are you using condoms as well?," asked the doctor.

"No, at least not consistently," Grace answered, somewhat embarrassed.

"Does your partner have any history of herpes or other sexually transmitted infections?," asked Dr. Chen.

Grace swallowed. How could she admit that she hadn't had the guts to even tell Miguel about her sore, much less ask if he had any diseases? Sitting here, it was hard to believe that she could have had sex with someone without knowing everything about his past. She had initially insisted on condoms to cover that possibility, but a few times there weren't any handy, and they had had sex anyway. "Um, not that I'm aware of."

Dr. Chen looked up at that response but didn't comment. "Okay. Last month, when you first noticed the sore, did you feel sick at all or have any fever?," asked the doctor.

Grace replied that she had been so busy and tired from studying that she didn't recall being particularly ill, just extremely uncomfortable from the sore.

"Have you put any creams or over-the-counter ointments on the sore?"

"No."

"All right, then. Let's go ahead and take a look," said Dr. Chen, setting down her chart.

Grace took a deep breath as she leaned backward and began to scoot down the exam table. Yet another fresh wave of tears filled her eyes. "Please let me be wrong," she thought. "Please, please, please. I don't want an infection that is going to stay with me the rest of my life. Maybe I'm just being paranoid." After all, "medical student disease" was a common phenomenon among her classmates these days. Whatever disease they studied, several students began to believe that they were suffering from it. Of course, the common symptoms of many infections, like fatigue, headache, weight gain, or bowel changes, were occurring in every student from the stress of school, but...

"Okay, let's get your feet in these stirrups," said the doctor, pulling out and positioning the hidden metal supports at the base of the exam table. Dr. Chen's voice snapped Grace back to reality, and she placed her feet one at a time in the sock-covered stirrups. She felt the heat from the lamp and squeezed her eyes shut. "Just relax," the doctor instructed.

Grace almost laughed. She had to remember never to tell a patient that. How could anyone possibly relax at this point?

"Here?," inquired Dr. Chen, pointing to the sore. "Is this the spot you were talking about?" Grace opened her eyes and looked down. "Yes, that's it. What do you think?"

"Well, I'm sorry, but honestly, it does look like herpes. What I'm seeing is a cluster of about five little blisters, which are starting to crust over, and the edge is bright red. I'm going to do a viral culture to confirm it, but I think we should start treatment while we're waiting for the results."

Grace's heart sank. Dr. Chen reached for a metal instrument that Grace recognized as a speculum and inserted it deftly, saying, "Grace, I'm going to take a quick look at your cervix and make sure there aren't any additional lesions inside."

Grace tried to focus on the memory of one of her classmates using a speculum as a duck puppet, opening and closing the "bills" of the tool and quacking. Before long, the doctor had removed the instrument and was pressing around the outside portion of Grace's pelvis.

"You have some enlarged lymph nodes down here, did you realize that? Feel right here." Grace obediently reached down and was surprised to feel a tender knot in her right groin. "Okay, you can slide back and sit up. Let me step out while you get dressed. I'll be right back in to finish talking with you."

Dazed, Grace went through the motions of getting dressed. Herpes. The "gift that keeps on giving," as one of her classmates so eloquently put it. "Oh my gosh, how am I going to tell Miguel? Actually, he's the one who had better be apologizing to me, since I've never had an outbreak before. What a jerk. I'm going to strangle him when I..."

A quick knock interrupted her thoughts. "Are you dressed?," asked Dr. Chen.

"Yes, come in," replied Grace.

"I'm going to talk to you as though you were not a medical student, and just give you my standard speech so I'm sure that I told you everything, without assuming that you know all about this, okay?"

Grace felt on the verge of tears again, so she simply nodded in agreement.

"All right. Your sores do look like herpes. In a couple of days, we'll get results from the tests that I took, and then we'll know for certain." Dr. Chen stopped a moment to hand Grace a tissue and then continued. "We abbreviate herpes simplex virus as HSV, not to be confused with HPV, the wart virus, nor with HIV, which causes

AIDS. With herpes, there are two types, aptly named herpes simplex virus type one and type two, or abbreviated simply as HSV-1 and HSV-2. Initially we thought all oral herpes sores were type one, and all genital lesions were type two. Oral herpes infections are still HSV-1 the vast majority of the time, and research shows that somewhere between fifty and eighty percent of people living in the United States have been infected with oral herpes by the age of twenty, *whether they actively break out with sores or not*."

"Do you mean sexually active adults, or all adults?," Grace asked.

"All adults. Much of HSV-1 is transmitted within families by kissing or sharing cups or utensils with infected adults in the home. Anyway, given the frequency of oral herpes, it shouldn't surprise you to learn that we have been seeing an increase in the number of cases of genital herpes that are actually type one, transmitted through oral sex. Studies show that the majority of newly diagnosed genital herpes are HSV type one. Many young people abstain from genital sex in the hope of avoiding sexually transmittable infections, and then, ironically, they end up here with genital herpes as the result of receiving oral sex from a partner who was infected with oral herpes. Also, while many people use condoms consistently for genital intercourse, fewer people realize that they should use condoms for oral sex."

Grace nodded to show she was listening, but her head was swimming with questions. Did Miguel know he had herpes? Why didn't she insist on condoms? Why didn't *he* insist on condoms? How could they have been so careless?

Dr. Chen pressed on earnestly, "Regardless of the type of herpes, we have antiviral drugs that really help a great deal. Unfortunately, we don't have anything yet that completely eradicates the infection, but at least the medications help outbreaks go away more quickly. We're going to get you started on one today, in fact. There are several different brands, but they work roughly the same way. The prescription I sent electronically to your pharmacy is for valacyclovir, five hundred milligrams, and you will take one pill twice per day for three days. The medicine is usually very well tolerated, but some people experience some stomach upset or headache. To begin with, you'll just take the medicine whenever you have an outbreak.

It's important to start the medicine as soon as you notice anything. Many people have a sensation of burning, tingling, or itching before they actually break out with the blisters. If you do get that, be sure to start taking the medicine at the first hint of your symptoms. The sooner into the outbreak that you start taking the medicine, the shorter the duration of the outbreak."

"So if I start the medicine right away, how long do you think I'll have these blisters?"

"Since this is not your first outbreak, I would expect that these will only last around four or five days, but everyone is different," the doctor replied.

"How frequently do you think I'll break out?," Grace asked, her voice tremulous.

Dr. Chen frowned. "I wish I could tell you 'infrequently,' but I have to say that with the mental and physical stress of med school, I would bet that you may have frequent outbreaks the first year or two. You've already established an early pattern of breaking out around your period, right?"

"In retrospect, yes. But this is only my second occurrence."

"Well, if it turns out that you are having frequent outbreaks, I think we should put you on suppressive therapy, instead of just treating eruptions."

"What does that mean?," asked Grace.

"We put you on a once-a-day dose as prevention, rather than simply taking the pills only when you break out. With this daily preventive dosing, we hope the herpes virus will stay dormant and you won't have as many outbreaks," said Dr. Chen.

"Why don't we just do that from the beginning, then?," asked Grace.

"I guess we could. To be honest, the main reason I wouldn't suggest it right now is the expense. If your finances are like mine were during medical school, it would be tough to justify the cost of daily therapy until you see a true pattern of how often you're going to break out," she answered.

"How much money are we talking about?," asked Grace.

"It's hard to say because there are so many variables, like if you are paying cash versus using insurance, and whether you are okay with generic medications. Without any insurance, the name brand anti-herpes drugs that you only have to take twice a day for three to five days can cost around sixty dollars per treatment. If you were taking it daily for suppressive treatment, that could be about two hundred dollars per month."

"Oh my gosh—that's a lot of money," gasped Grace. "But I have the student health insurance, and I am pretty sure I only have a co-pay with my prescriptions. I think it's like fifteen dollars if it's generic, and thirty-five if it's name brand."

"You're lucky—with my insurance, the co-pay for prescriptions starts at thirty bucks for the generic. Anyway, the cost all depends on which drugs are on your insurance company's formulary."

"Not to be clueless, but what is a formulary?," asked Grace.

"Sorry, I should have explained. A formulary is a list of the specific medications that an insurance company decides to provide its clients. Every insurance company makes its own contracts with the drug companies, so the amount of your co-pay depends on which medications are on the preferred list for your company this year. Acyclovir, which is the generic name for Zovirax, is the oldest anti-herpes medication, so it is the least expensive, but you have to take it three times per day. Valacyclovir, which has the same active ingredient as Valtrex, is a newer generic medication which should be taken twice daily. Famciclovir is the most recent herpes medication to go generic—its name brand is Famvir. I am fine if you want to decide which drug you want to take based on what your insurance company says about pricing," said Dr. Chen.

"Is it possible for you to give me samples of these three medications so I can see if there's any difference in side effects?," asked Grace.

"No, I'm sorry. Since these drugs all have generic equivalents now, we don't get samples anymore. The drug companies just tend to leave samples of the newest medicines," she replied.

"Really? I didn't realize that doctors didn't get samples for all types of medications," Grace responded. "Our family doctor always gave us samples when we saw her."

"In our practice, we no longer accept any type of drug samples," replied Dr. Chen. "Although I will be the first to admit that I loved being able to hand my patients medications to start right away, we want to be sure that as clinicians we are not being biased in our drug choices based on overt or subliminal perks from the drug companies. The university's policy is that we allow pharmaceutical reps to talk to us about their medications, but we no longer accept any type of gifts—meals, free pens, or even patient handouts that include drug brand names."

Dr. Chen shrugged her shoulders, then went back to talking about herpes. "Anyway, you should know that some people are so sensitive that they cannot even wear jeans for a year or so because anything rubbing in the area causes an outbreak. Other people have one or two outbreaks and then don't have another for a very long time. The herpes virus likes to pick one nerve pathway to erupt from, so people tend to break out in the same spot, or at least on the same side in roughly the same spot, each time."

Dr. Chen grimaced slightly as she went on: "In my clinical experience, women have the worse end of the deal. Periods are a very common trigger for outbreaks, so obviously that alone makes it worse for females. People under a lot of stress of any kind—nutritional, sleep, physical, or mental stress—tend to have more frequent outbreaks. We'll just have to see how you do, and how you tolerate the medicine, before we can make an intelligent decision about how to treat you. Does that make sense?"

"Yes, I guess so," agreed Grace.

Dr. Chen was entering notes on her computer as she spoke. Grace waited until the doctor appeared to be finished with her typing, and then asked the question that had been bothering her most: "Is there anything else I need to know about herpes? I mean, can this affect me down the road when I want to have kids?"

Dr. Chen sat back from the computer. "Well," she replied, "it really shouldn't affect your ability to conceive. Other STIs, like chlamydia and gonorrhea, can certainly cause scarring of the fallopian tubes and lead to infertility, but we really don't see that with herpes. The main issue with pregnancy and herpes is about delivery. If you have an active lesion when it is time to deliver, we do C-sections instead of vaginal deliveries. Does that answer your question?"

Grace nodded yes.

"And speaking of other STIs, I also did a test on you during the pelvic exam that checks for chlamydia and gonorrhea. Any time you have one STI, we always check for others. Unfortunately, STIs seem to like to travel in packs, as we say. When you get one, you frequently get another at the same time. So, I suggest that we draw blood and screen for HIV. You'll need to sign a separate consent form for that, by the way. We should have the results from all your tests in a couple of days. Our nurse will call you when we've got them back. Do you have any other questions about herpes in general?," the doctor asked.

"Yes, one more that I can think of right now. Is there anything, uh, holistic, or whatever, that I can do to make the herpes better? You know, like take extra vitamins?," Grace asked.

"I'm glad you asked that. If you get on the Internet or look in any health food store, you'll find a million remedies that claim to prevent herpes outbreaks. The only successful one that I'm aware of from my own clinical experience with patients over the years is taking lysine daily, which seems to help prevent outbreaks," she said.

"Lysine—that's an amino acid, isn't it? How does that work?," asked Grace.

Dr. Chen shrugged. "I don't think anyone knows exactly, but I can tell you that I do have some patients that swear by it. They take one hundred milligrams per day to help prevent outbreaks, then triple the dose during any flare-ups."

"Got it," said Grace. "I guess my only other questions are about transmission. When am I contagious? Just when I can see or feel the blisters?"

"No. Unfortunately, doctors used to think that herpes was only contagious during outbreaks. Now we know that you can shed the virus, and therefore infect someone else, even when you cannot see or feel anything. So, ultimately, you really need to use condoms from now on, because they reduce the risk of transmitting herpes."

"Only reduce the risk?," Grace questioned.

"Yes, because condoms cannot cover all the areas where the virus can be transmitted."

"So, I'll need to use condoms forever?"

"Or at least until you're married and trying to conceive."

"And if my future husband doesn't have herpes? What are the chances that I'll pass it on to him if at that point, presumably years from now, if I'm no longer having many or, I hope, any outbreaks?," asked Grace tentatively.

"Again, I don't have an exact statistic for you. I can tell you that some long-term sexual partners of people with herpes never break out, so transmission is not one hundred percent, anyway," replied Dr. Chen.

"Well, that's good, but I guess now I'm obligated to tell anyone that I'm intimate with that I've got herpes, even if I plan to always use condoms."

"Yes," affirmed Dr. Chen. "Unfortunately, many people are either too embarrassed or just plain dishonest, and they pass on all kinds of sexually transmitted infections because they don't tell their significant others. I know it's hard to share that kind of information, but it's really important."

The doctor stood up and handed Grace her paperwork so she could check out. "You should be hearing from us by the end of the week with your test results. Let's hope we won't need to treat anything else, but if we do, we'll bring you back in and take care of it. If you have any more problems, or if you start having frequent outbreaks, come back in and we'll change you over to daily therapy."

"Okay, thanks," said Grace. She had actually begun feeling a little better during their conversation, until the doctor mentioned treating anything else. Anything else? As if this weren't bad enough. Tears welled up in her eyes as she gathered her purse and coat. Herpes. I've got to tell Miguel I've got herpes. No, not I—*we've* got herpes. Oh great, this really was going to be hard. Should she yell at him for giving her herpes? Her heart sank. It really didn't matter. Ultimately what mattered to Grace was that she had genital herpes, now and forever. She'd just have to get past it. "Maybe," she thought sadly, "maybe this will make me a better doctor. A little more compassionate, less judgmental... Oh man, this was not how I expected to learn about sexually transmitted infections."

2: Justin

SUNDAY MORNING TRAINING RIDES were always the best. Few cars, clear blue skies, birds screeching greetings, and Lake Austin glistening in the early light under the Loop 360 bridge presented an amazing backdrop for the cycling group as they drafted behind one another. Justin's legs burned as he powered up the long, steep hill, sweat pouring down his forehead and stinging his eyes. The adrenaline surge kicked his heart into high gear, and it raced hard to fuel his screaming legs. Justin imagined himself competing in the Tour de France, pulling for his team as crowds cheered him on. As his fantasy played in his head, Justin stood up on his pedals, pumping his legs madly for the final hundred meters; he crested the hill physically exhausted but emotionally charged up with the sheer joy of the ride.

As he reached the top, Justin dropped back onto the saddle of his bike and unexpectedly winced in pain. It was as though a Mack truck had run over him, instantly deflating the joy that had welled up in his chest. "Not again," he agonized.

At five foot eleven, with a hundred and seventy pounds of wiry muscle and virtually no body fat, he looked to be the very picture of health. Justin's lopsided smile, deep blue eyes, and dark brown hair completed the all-American image. Justin *was* in excellent physical condition, with one exception. Justin had genital herpes.

When Justin had first arrived at the university, he was amazed at how easily and casually his female classmates offered oral sex at parties, especially if there was alcohol involved. Among his high school friends, only a few lucky guys had girlfriends who were willing to go down on them. At his first few college parties, however, Justin was surprised to learn that doing shots, grinding, making out, and getting head seemed to be the full party package. Although he had chosen not to have "real" sex yet, Justin had received oral sex from several different coeds. When he developed his first infection, Justin initially thought he had the flu: he had awakened with a fever, body aches, and a headache. However, the next day, he also developed amazingly painful blisters covering the right side of the tip of his penis. Justin was mortified when he received the diagnosis of herpes at the university health center later that week.

Over the next few semesters, Justin dated casually, but avoided physical intimacy. He wasn't attracted enough to any of the women to make it worth suffering through the embarrassment of explaining that he had herpes. It was far easier to stay superficial, hanging around in groups more than dating exclusively. At least, that had been the case until now.

Justin smiled at Kayla as he walked his bike over to his car. Kayla's electric-blue and purple biking shirt reflected her vibrant personality as it showed off her petite athletic figure. She was twenty, the same age as Justin. Kayla's lightly freckled face was sweaty, and her braided long brown hair was messed up from her helmet, but Justin still thought she looked great.

"That was an awesome ride. I didn't think I was going to make it up that last hill though," Kayla said, lifting her bike onto the rack behind Justin's.

"No kidding," Justin replied. "My legs feel like rubber. How about yours?"

"Well, let's just say that I'd rather grab some banana pancakes than go for a run," Kayla laughed.

"Okay, then let's head over to Magnolia Café," suggested Justin. Seeing that Kayla's water bottle had fallen off her bike and rolled to the edge of the parking area, he walked over to grab it for her. As he headed toward the curb, the burning and tingling in his crotch that had started on the ride began to intensify.

Kayla pointed at his legs, saying, "Justin, you weren't kidding about your legs. It looks like you're limping. Are you all right?"

Justin flushed with embarrassment. He realized that he must have been holding his hips off to the side to relieve some of the pressure on his groin. Thank goodness his face was already red and sweaty from the ride, so Kayla didn't notice the difference. For a split second, he thought of telling her the truth and just getting it out in the open. Instead, he exaggerated his limp, and in an old man's voice croaked, "Ah, I'm just getting to be too old to ride with cute young things like you. You've crippled me for life." Justin staggered back to the car, and he and Kayla drove off to breakfast.

A few days later, Justin was able to get an appointment to see Dr. Dillon, one of the doctors at the health center on campus.

"So, Justin, what's bothering you today?," asked the doctor.

Justin saw no point in beating around the bush. "Dr. Dillon, as you know, I've had herpes for nearly two years now," he said, pointing to his crotch to indicate which kind of herpes. "I'm really frustrated with these outbreaks," he blurted.

"How often are you getting them?," inquired Dr. Dillon.

"At least once or twice every semester," Justin answered.

"Do you have one now?," the doctor asked.

"Yes, but really that's not my point," Justin said.

"Okay, then what is your concern?," the doctor countered.

"Well, I'm trying to be healthy. I know that when I'm run down, I break out worse and more often. I'm clear that I need to have regular sleep and eat well, but you know that's not always a choice as a student."

"I disagree. I'm not saying it's easy, but it *is* technically a choice. What's your major?," asked Dr. Dillon.

"Architecture," answered Justin. "When our projects are due, our groups frequently work 'round the clock the last few days."

"Living on pizza and caffeine, no doubt," added Dr. Dillon, with a grin.

"Well, yes," said Justin defensively. "I get it that finals and project deadlines are going to trigger herpes. I just thought that by now, after two years, it would kind of... go away. How much longer do you think I'm going to have to deal with this?"

"Justin, you know we don't have a cure for herpes yet."

"Yes, but usually, doesn't it stop breaking out after a while?"

"Well, in some patients, it does. In others, the outbreaks may continue for decades, and we don't yet know why it affects people so differently," shrugged Dr. Dillon.

"I guess I'm just lucky then," said Justin sarcastically.

"You're certainly not the worst case I've ever seen, Justin." Dr. Dillon flipped through the chart, looking at previous notes. "You know, I've offered you suppressive therapy before, but you chose not to take it, so I guess it hasn't been that bad, right?"

"It's not that simple. Generally, I feel pretty healthy, and it just seems counterintuitive to take a medication every day of my life. Do we really know what risks there are from the medicine?," asked Justin.

Dr. Dillon leaned back in his chair. "In all my years of practice, I've never seen any serious complications from the anti-herpes drugs. They are generally very well tolerated. Occasionally, people get some nausea or headache, but it's hard to say if that is coming from the drug or actually from the recurrence of herpes. I don't know off the top of my head what the manufacturers of the drug list as the side effects. I just know what I hear complaints about. Let's see." He pulled out his phone and clicked on an app. "Famvir, famciclovir, lists these short-term complaints as possible side effects: headache—13.5 percent; migraine—0.6 percent; nausea—2.5 percent; diarrhea—4.9 percent; vomiting—1.2 percent; and fatigue—0.6 percent."

"And you wonder why I don't want to take it every day?," charged Justin. "What about some of the other medicines that I see ads for? Are they better?"

"In my clinical experience, they all have a similar side-effect profile. Also, remember, even placebos are listed as causing headaches, for example, at over five percent. There may be studies that show one drug might be slightly more effective than the others, but mainly it's a matter of patient preference because of how often you have to take the pills or individual side effects. I see your point, but honestly, I rarely have people complain about the medicine causing problems. Usually if they have a complaint, it's about the cost." Dr. Dillon looked expectantly at Justin. "So what do you think? Shall I send the pharmacy a prescription?," he asked, hands poised over his keyboard.

Justin sighed. "Look, I don't mean to be a pain, but I'm not sure. I've got some more questions, if you don't mind."

Dr. Dillon pushed back from his computer and swiveled his chair to face Justin directly, saying, "Fire away."

"Okay. One thing is, I love to cycle. I've tried a bunch of different sports, but biking is the only thing that I really enjoy and can do consistently. Do you think I'm making the herpes worse with biking?," asked Justin.

"Well, I imagine the combination of the tight biking shorts plus the friction against the saddle might aggravate your herpes. It's certainly not the ideal choice for you. Why don't you try running or, better yet, swimming?," Dr. Dillon suggested.

"I tore up my right knee snow skiing last spring break, and it swells up every time I run, so that's out. Swimming is okay, but it's not terribly convenient. It just takes up too much time to get to the pool or down to the lake to swim."

"Again, it's about choices. What do you think? Have you noticed more outbreaks since you started riding?," inquired Dr. Dillon.

"I'm not sure if it causes outbreaks, but if I already have the blisters and I go for any ride longer than thirty or forty minutes, they'll take forever to go away," Justin answered.

"Makes sense, I suppose. Why don't you try taking the medicine daily for a few months? Let's see if that will prevent the outbreaks altogether." He again turned back to the keyboard and started to type.

As the doctor entered in his prescription, Justin realized he had more questions. What he really wanted to ask was: When and how in the world should he tell Kayla about his herpes? Dr. Dillon was nice enough, but today he seemed kind of in a hurry. Justin decided on a different tack. "Dr. Dillon, I have a new girlfriend. We haven't, um, done anything yet. I certainly don't want to give her this. If we decide to have sex, what are the chances that she would get herpes from me if I use a condom?"

"Statistics show that in an exclusive relationship, if you completely abstain from sex during any outbreaks, and consistently use a condom when you have sex in between flare-ups, she will have a ten percent risk of developing herpes at the end of a year. It's not zero, because condoms don't cover all the areas where the virus can be spread. Just so you know, an uninfected woman is at higher risk of getting herpes from an infected male than vice versa," rattled off Dr. Dillon.

"Why's that?"

"During sex, a woman gets microscopic abrasions in her vagina that make her more susceptible to infection. By the way, from your question, I'm assuming your new girlfriend doesn't have genital herpes. Do you know if she gets the mouth sores of oral herpes?," asked Dr. Dillon.

"I've never seen one on her, but we haven't had a discussion about it yet. Does it matter?," wondered Justin.

"Yes, actually, it does. If she already has oral herpes, that ten percent risk number I told you is accurate. If, however, she doesn't have antibodies to any type of herpes, her chance of getting herpes from you goes up to about thirty-two percent."

"So you're basically telling me that I should hope that Kayla has oral herpes. Great. That's what got me into this in the first place. What about beyond a year? Just for the sake of discussion, say we got married. Is she guaranteed to get herpes from me? Obviously, if we wanted to have kids, we wouldn't be using a condom then," said Justin.

"Well, there are some long-term couples in which one partner has herpes, and the other one seems to be free of infection. Perhaps they have a mild case that they're unaware of, or they just have great antibodies. Either way, it does happen, but we don't have enough long-term studies to give you a solid answer right now. What you really need to know is that you are contagious, whether or not you're having an outbreak. You definitely shed more virus immediately before, during, and after an outbreak, but it's thought that up to seventy percent of transmission occurs when people think they are not contagious," Dr. Dillon lectured.

"That doesn't make sense," muttered Justin, doing the math in his head.

"Think about it," said Dr. Dillon. "People are more careful, abstaining from sex when they feel symptoms like burning or itching before an outbreak, and certainly when they can see blisters, right? And that's when they shed the most virus so that's when potentially they're the most contagious."

"Okay," agreed Justin.

"But in between outbreaks, when there is no visible sign of herpes, people don't feel contagious, and they are intimate more often. So they are less contagious, but more sexually active, and therefore more infections are transmitted," clarified the doctor.

"I saw on a commercial that if you take this medicine every day, it's supposed to help decrease the chance that you can pass on the infection. Is that true?," inquired Justin.

"Yes, fortunately it is. Studies have proven that if you take suppressive daily valacyclovir, a herpes antiviral drug, it decreases the risk of passing on herpes to an uninfected partner by up to fifty percent."

"What about hot tubs? If I'm having an outbreak, so I'm shedding all this virus, can I give it to people if we all go hot tubbing together?," asked Justin.

Dr. Dillon laughed. "No. Don't be concerned about that. No hot tubs, toilet seats, or any other objects that people share purely externally can transmit herpes. This virus is not that hardy. It dies when the secretions carrying it dry up. Now, two people sharing sex toys could absolutely pass it on, but just hanging around other people is perfectly safe."

"No worries there," Justin replied. He sat for a moment, processing everything the doctor had said.

Dr. Dillon stood up. "Let me examine you quickly to make sure this is genital herpes. I know we've diagnosed it before, but let's just confirm it. Have you had any new sexual partners since your last visit?"

It was Justin's turn to laugh. "No, Dr. Dillon. I've actually never even had intercourse. I got this just from getting oral sex a few times. I can't imagine what else it could be—it's a clump of small blisters in the same spot where they always show up."

Dr. Dillon motioned for Justin to lie back. "Let's just take a look to be sure." It took only a few seconds, and then Dr. Dillon's confirmation came in a sympathetic tone. "Yes, Justin, you have a very typical lesion. See here, the base is bright red, and your cluster of blisters is already scabbing over." He sat on his stool and scanned through Justin's chart again.

"What are you looking for?," asked Justin.

"I'm looking to see if we ever checked your antibodies to see what type of herpes you have. Classically, herpes type one used to be the main source of oral herpes, and type two was the cause of genital lesions, but now it's closer to an equal distribution."

"What difference does it make?," wondered Justin.

"I guess it's a bit academic," said Dr. Dillon, "but usually type one herpes in the genital region doesn't cause as many outbreaks as you've dealt with, so I was curious." He paused for a moment, then added, "Also, I was thinking about your new girlfriend. If you know what type of herpes you have, she can be tested to see if she has antibodies. Most adults have antibodies to at least one type of herpes, and if she has antibodies to the same type that you have, she'll be somewhat protected."

A wave of cautious optimism began to creep over Justin. "Okay, then, if it's not in my chart, let's test me and find out. I don't remember anyone ever telling me which type I have. I thought since it was in my crotch, I automatically had type two. I never thought about where it came from. So, if you have type one, for example, you can still catch type two, but it doesn't matter where in your body you or the other person has herpes. Is that right?"

Dr. Dillon nodded. "That's more or less correct. You 'catch' herpes only by direct contact with it, so in that sense, it does matter where you or your partner have it. Typically, a person infected with one type of herpes in their genitals will not get a new genital infection of herpes simplex virus, even if they are exposed to a different type. Also, if you have type one herpes in your genital area, and your girlfriend has type one herpes in her mouth, you will not develop a new spot of herpes if she performs oral sex on you. Does that make sense?"

Justin nodded, still absorbing the information.

Dr. Dillon continued, "However, if you have type one genital herpes, and she has type two oral herpes, you potentially could catch a new infection. The most likely place for it to show up would be in your mouth, from kissing her."

"And if, instead, I have type two down there?," quizzed Justin.

"Type two herpes seems to produce a more protective antibody response. If you have type two herpes in your genitals, you are often protected against developing a new type one infection anywhere in your body," said Dr. Dillon.

"By saying 'often,' I assume you mean not one hundred percent," said Justin.

"Yes. Of course, no matter what, I recommend using a condom if you're having any kind of sex, to prevent spreading not only herpes but any other infection as well. If you're thinking about having sex with your girlfriend, I'd advise that both of you be fully tested for all sexually transmitted infections. We can do that today, if you'd like," advised Dr. Dillon.

"What else could I possibly have, if I've never had real sex?," asked Justin.

"Well, we know you've had enough exposure to get herpes, which means you could potentially have another infection. It sounds like you are certainly at a lower risk, but it's not zero. I'd like to check you for everything, including gonorrhea, chlamydia, HIV, hepatitis C, and syphilis. You're immunized against hepatitis B, so at least we don't need to worry about that one. I didn't see any genital warts, lice, or other obvious lesions. Look, it's far easier to have an honest conversation with your girlfriend if you can assure one another that you have been tested for all sexually transmittable infections." Dr. Dillon stood up, handing Justin a lab slip. "Most infections are not as obvious as your herpes. Lots of them don't even have any symptoms. If you are going to be sexually intimate, whether you think it's 'real sex' or not, wear a condom every time, and talk to your partner about all this before you're in a situation where talking isn't your priority. I sent the pharmacy a prescription for a three-month supply of valacyclovir, which is the generic form of the name brand Valtrex. Why don't you follow up with me at the end of the prescription and let me know if it stopped the outbreaks, okay?"

"Sure, that seems reasonable. Thanks," Justin replied.

Justin went to the lab and had his blood drawn, then stopped at the pharmacy to get his medicine. He still wasn't sure how long he was going to take it, but it seemed reasonable to give it a try.

A few days went by, and Justin had no side effects that he was aware of from the medicine. His lesions had cleared up enough that he felt okay to bike ride again, so he texted Kayla and set up a Saturday morning biking date, preceded by a Friday night Italian dinner.

"Gotta love carbo-loading," murmured Justin, swallowing a mouthful of pasta.

"Where do you want to ride tomorrow?," asked Kayla, wiping the tomato sauce from her mouth. She grimaced when she touched the corner of her mouth. "Oh man, I think I'm getting another cold sore," she complained.

Startled, Justin leaned across the table, staring intently at her mouth. "Do you have herpes?," he blurted out. He was partly dismayed, but at the same time partly relieved.

Kayla pulled back, her hand protectively covering her mouth. "Yuck—herpes?" Her face contorted in an appalled look. "No! I just get these cold sores when I'm stressed out. With finals around the corner, it wouldn't surprise me one is popping up. Why would you ask if this is herpes? Do you have herpes?"

Here it was, the moment of truth. But the look of disgust on Kayla's face as she said "herpes" was too much. If Kayla thought a mouth ulcer was "yuck," what would she think if he told her he had sores in his crotch? Justin's brain raced wildly, wanting to be honest but fearful it was too early in their relationship to broach the whole topic.

"No, no, I don't get sores in my mouth," Justin said, skirting the complete truth. "It's no big deal anyway, I was just curious. I read somewhere that most cold sores are herpes. You see those commercials on television all the time now, so I was just going to say you might want to check with your doctor." Quickly, he switched topics. "Anyway, back to the ride. I thought maybe we'd head over to Bastrop and bike in the pine woods tomorrow. I hear there are some great hills to conquer over there, if you're up for it," he challenged.

"Bet I can beat you up the last hill," Kayla retorted, and happily chatted on about the weather expected in the morning.

Justin realized this conversation might come back to haunt him some day, but technically, he had been honest. And he was nearly certain that what Kayla said was "just a cold sore" was actually herpes. Justin's test results were not back yet, but since he knew for certain that he had contracted his genital herpes from oral sex, the odds were in their favor that he and Kayla had the same type of herpes. Justin promised himself that the next time the subject came up, he would tell Kayla the full story about herpes, including how he ended up with genital herpes from oral sex. For now, he'd be content to get to know Kayla better, and perhaps learn more about her past experiences. Justin glanced at her lips again, only barely able to see the sore that was forming just above the corner of her mouth.

"Better not do any kissing tonight," he thought, startling himself with what seemed a bit of a double standard.

"Wait," Justin told himself. "I'm not being unreasonable. I just don't want to get oral herpes, now that I understand about the different types." The more he pondered it, the more he was sincerely worried about catching oral herpes. Justin knew that he couldn't go back to kissing Kayla until they knew which type she had, which meant having a full-blown conversation about sexually transmittable infections.

"Hey there, are you listening? I was asking if you wanted a taste of my tiramisu." Kayla interrupted his internal debate as she extended a piece of her dessert on a fork.

Justin internally recoiled but simply said, "No, thanks. I'm too stuffed to manage even one more bite."

"Okay, but your loss is my... weight gain." Kayla laughed, making a show of savoring the dessert.

Justin couldn't help but smile at her antics, his mood rebounding. Kayla's bubbly enthusiasm was irresistible. "She's worth it," he silently affirmed, reaching to squeeze her hand. Cold sore or not, herpes or not, Kayla was awesome, and Justin was ready to move forward.

"Like you need to worry about your weight! Besides, we'll burn off a zillion calories in the hills. Cheers to tomorrow," he concluded, raising his glass in a toast.

facts

Herpes Simplex Virus (HSV) Fact Sheet

What is it?

- Herpes is a DNA virus.
- There are two strains: type 1 and type 2.
- Type 1 more commonly occurs in the mouth, and type 2 more often in the genitals, but both can occur in either location.
- One person can be infected with both types.

How common is it?

- Estimates vary, but between 50% and 90% of adults have oral herpes by age 50.

- 25% of adults have genital herpes, but up to 90% of them are unaware of it.

How do you get it?

- Through direct skin contact with an infected area.
- From secretions infected with HSV: saliva, vaginal secretions, or semen (including on shared utensils or toothbrushes).

Where on your body do you get it?

- Most often on a mucosal surface: the mouth or genital skin.
- Less often on any skin surface, such as arms or legs, unless the skin is broken (for example, if it has been bitten or scratched).

How do I know if I have it?

- Many people are asymptomatic, so the only way to know if you have been infected is through a blood test.
- Blood tests check for antibodies to HSV-1 and HSV-2.
- HSV DNA testing or a herpes culture taken by swabbing a new lesion can confirm herpes infection.

What does it look like?

- A small red bump or blister or a cluster of bumps or blisters on a bright red base.

What does it feel like?

- Many people feel itching, burning, or tingling before they see any lesions.

- Blisters may be extremely painful or mildly annoying.
- Nearby lymph nodes (in the neck or groin) may swell and ache.
- Especially with the initial outbreak, additional symptoms may include headache, muscle aches, stiff neck, sore throat, fever, and other flu-like symptoms.

How long does it last?

- Initial outbreak lasts 1–2 weeks on average.
- Recurrent outbreaks last 3–7 days.

Can it be cured?

- No. Once infected, you will always have the virus.

What is the treatment?

- Antiviral medicines, such as acyclovir (Zovirax), famciclovir (Famvir), and valacyclovir (Valtrex), can reduce the duration and intensity of an outbreak if taken as soon as you are aware of symptoms, preferably before blisters even form.
- Medicines can be taken daily to prevent frequent recurrences.

How about alternative therapies?

- Wearing loose clothes can allow the sores to dry out.
- Reducing stress can help prevent outbreaks.
- Some patients may find that taking daily lysine supplements decreases the frequency or intensity of flare-ups, but there are no large clinical studies confirming this practice.

Are there long-term consequences of herpes?

- HSV does not cause scarring unless there is a secondary infection from a bacteria (like a staph or strep infection caused by scratching).
- New HSV infections during pregnancy are harmful to the fetus, and HSV can infect a child passing through the birth canal. Most expectant mothers who have herpes choose to have a Cesarean section to decrease risk of transmission.

When are you contagious?

- Always!
- Herpes is most infective immediately before, during, and after an outbreak.

How do I avoid getting genital herpes?

- Abstinence from sexual intimacy (direct genital contact: oral, vaginal, and/or anal sex) is the only 100% effective prevention.
- Males should always wear a condom when they receive oral sex, which protects both parties: the receiver from getting herpes transmitted from the giver's mouth, and the giver's mouth from any STIs carried by the receiver.
- Condom use decreases transmission but is not totally effective because the virus can be shed outside of the area that condoms cover.
- Use new condoms for each partner with any shared sex toys or, preferably, do not share sex toys.

If I have herpes, how do I avoid giving it to my partner?

- Daily valacyclovir (suppressive treatment) can reduce viral shedding and therefore reduce transmission of herpes.
- Abstinence during outbreaks paired with condom use in between outbreaks reduces the transmission of herpes to an uninfected partner.

Does herpes transmission occur in homosexual partners?

- Oral-genital transmission can occur regardless of gender.
- Shared sex toys can transmit the herpes virus.
- Herpes can be transmitted during anal intercourse.

Frequently Asked Questions

➤ **Can you catch herpes from a toilet seat?**
No. The virus dies quickly outside the body, especially when it gets dry.

➤ **Are most oral "cold sores" from vitamin deficiencies?**
No. Most cold sores are herpes simplex.

➤ **Can you catch genital herpes from oral sex?**
Yes. This is a frequent source of transmission.

➤ **If you can't see or feel any sores, are you contagious?**
Yes. If you have herpes, you are always potentially contagious.

➤ **If you develop herpes in a monogamous relationship, is your partner cheating?**
Not necessarily, because it can take weeks, months, or years after exposure until you first notice an outbreak.

Additional Information

American College of Obstetricians and Gynecologists
PO Box 70620
Washington, DC 20024-9998
1-800-673-8444
www.acog.org/publications/patient_education/bp054.cfm

Centers for Disease Control and Prevention
1600 Clifton Road
Atlanta, GA 30329-4027
1-800-CDC-INFO (1-800-232-4636), 1-888-232-6348 (TTY)
www.cdc.gov/std/Herpes/default.htm

The Good News about the Bad News: Herpes: Everything You Need to Know by Terri Warren, RN, NP (Oakland, CA: New Harbinger, 2009)

MedlinePlus
US National Library of Medicine
8600 Rockville Pike
Bethesda, MD 20894
1-888-FIND-NLM (1-888-346-3656) or 301-594-5983
www.nlm.nih.gov/medlineplus/herpessimplex.html

National Herpes Resource Center and Hotline
American Sexual Health Association
PO Box 13827
Research Triangle Park, NC 27709
919-361-8400
www.ashasexualhealth.org/

HUMAN PAPILLOMA VIRUS

3: Chase

CHASE GLANCED AROUND THE waiting room. Some people smiled and nodded at him with recognition. At six foot four, two hundred and ten pounds, with bright red hair and freckles, Chase tended to stick out in a crowd. "Oh great," he thought. "Of all the times to be recognized, this was not a good one." This year had been absolutely amazing. It was his senior year of high school, and he had finally been picked over his long-term rival and buddy, Dalton, to be the first-string quarterback. Although the first couple of games had been a bit shaky, by the third game Chase had found his groove, and the Chargers were easily dominating their opponents each week. His picture had been plastered across the front page of the local paper, and now everyone was speculating about which college recruiters were after him.

"I think they know my football star son," Chase's mother whispered to him with pride. Chase groaned in response. His mom continued, "Don't worry. I'm sure Dr. Morris will get you fixed up in time for this Friday, honey. Can you believe the scouts from UCLA are coming to the game?" Chase's mom was a UCLA alumna, and she would love nothing more than to see her son playing for her alma mater. "Besides, Dr. Morris is a Bruin too, so I know she'll want you in top form this weekend. Do you think she'll be wearing her blue-and-gold scrubs today?"

Chase smiled. He'd been seeing Dr. Morris since grade school. He had outgrown the sticker and lollipop rewards at the end of the visits, but he still enjoyed seeing her. Dr. Morris bounded with energy and always made him laugh. Most of her staff supported the other local university and football powerhouse, the USC Trojans, but Dr. Morris was always optimistic that her Bruins would some day win the national championship. She had teased Chase for years that he would be just the quarterback to lead them to that victory.

Shifting nervously in his chair, Chase thought about explaining today's visit to the doctor. He must have made a face, because suddenly his mom's brow furrowed, and she asked him, "Does it hurt very much? I hope that giving you ibuprofen was the right thing to do."

"Honestly, it's really not that bad anymore, Mom," Chase said. "I mainly just want to be sure that I'm in good shape this week. I bet I won't even have to miss a practice."

"Chase?," Debbie, the nurse, stood at the door to the office, calling his name from the clipboard she held. Chase jumped up, waving his mom back.

"Uh, Mom, I'm fine by myself. Just wait out here, and I'll be right back." Chase's mother was already half out of her chair, ready to follow him.

"Okay, honey. If you'd rather see the doctor by yourself, I guess I'll wait here," she said with a martyred sigh. Chase let out his own sigh, one of relief, and was thankful that he had begun occasionally seeing Dr. Morris by himself a few years ago. Now his mom wouldn't be suspicious that anything was up.

His mother had insisted on driving him this morning, claiming her parental rights since he was leaving for college in six months, saying that she had a right to baby him as long as he lived at home. His dad had also offered to bring him, but Chase had quickly reassured both of them that the office visit was just a precaution. The nurse walked him down the familiar hallway, stopping at the scale to weigh him.

"That was some game you played Friday night," she said with a warm smile. "You're giving those cheerleaders lots of reasons to celebrate this year."

Chase grinned, saying, "Let's hope we do it again this weekend. This game will be much tougher."

"Well, we'll just have to make sure we've got you in perfect health by then. No pressure. After all, we've got four whole days 'til the next game." They both laughed as she led him into an exam room and motioned for him to sit on the exam table.

"Okay, Chase," Debbie said as she wrapped the blood pressure cuff around his arm. "So you pulled something in your groin Friday night?"

"Um, I guess that's what happened..." Chase's voice trailed off. At what point did he need to tell the truth? Did it matter what he said to the nurse, or could he just wait until Dr. Morris came in?

"How did it happen? Did it start hurting immediately after you were tackled, or did you not notice it until after the game?"

Chase felt his face flushing. "Uh... to be honest... I was embarrassed to tell the receptionist, but..." He bit his lip and swallowed hard.

"Chase." He looked up at the nurse. Debbie had worked at Dr. Morris's office since Chase was in middle school. She smiled gently, removing the cuff from his arm. "Don't worry. If there is something else you need to tell the doctor, remember we're here to take care of any problem you have—even if it's embarrassing. Do you feel comfortable telling me what's really going on?"

Chase wanted to just disappear. He tried to act like he was talking about something completely boring. "Well," he said, willing his voice to jump back down to the right octave, "I'm sure it's nothing, but I noticed a few bumps on my... uh... down there." He pointed at his crotch. "It seems like they're kind of multiplying, so I thought I'd better get it checked out. It's probably from my jock strap or something." His voice trailed off.

"It's okay, Chase, Dr. Morris will figure out what's going on, and she'll help you fix it. Please get undressed from the waist down, and you can put this sheet over yourself and sit on the end of the exam table. Dr. Morris will be in shortly." Debbie handed him the sheet and stepped out of the room.

Chase quickly shed his jeans and boxers and situated himself on the end of the table. He thought back to Saturday morning. He had been going through his usual postgame Saturday morning routine of soaking in a hot bath and letting his stiff muscles relax when he saw the bumps. A few weeks ago, he had noticed two small reddish bumps just below the head of his penis. They didn't itch or hurt, and he basically had ignored them and figured they would go away. Last weekend though, he was dismayed to see that there seemed to be a whole cluster of them, and they looked kind of wrinkly on top. Chase knew he had to see Dr. Morris and find out what was going on.

However, there was no way that he would tell his parents there was something growing on his penis. "Can you imagine what a torrent of questions that would set off?," Chase thought. His dad had been giving him monthly speeches about "the birds and the bees," which basically consisted of his father stammering around for a while and ending up saying, "Son, just be sure you use condoms. You don't want to get some girl pregnant and ruin both of your lives, not to mention your football career. Remember, sports are your ticket to a college education, and education"—here, Chase would join in and finish the sentence—"is your ticket to life." Other than that, his parents pretty much stayed out of his social life, though his mom had asked a bunch of questions when he and Sydney started hanging out together last summer.

Sydney babysat for her next-door neighbor's kids in the mornings. Chase and a few of his buddies mowed lawns, but they usually tried to finish their work by noon, before it got too hot. This left their afternoons free, and a big group got together most afternoons and evenings at the lake. Sydney's parents had a lake house with a boat, so that was the usual gathering place. Their friends were mainly jocks and cheerleaders, all of them filled with anticipation for their senior year. They loved skiing, wakeboarding, and just hanging out.

Within the group, there were several couples that were "serious." By midsummer, Chase was having sex with Sydney. Chase knew enough to use condoms, even though she was on the pill. Her parents thought she was taking the pill just to help with her periods, and she had told Chase that she was a virgin. They were committed to one another and talked of going to the same college. In fairness, Chase thought now, Sydney had talked much more about their future together, while he was more excited about the present.

Chase's parents had seemed relieved when he and Sydney broke up in August. They liked her well enough, but his mom was convinced that Sydney was trying to tie him down, and his dad was mainly worried that she would distract him from football practice. The truth was, when Sydney dumped Chase in August for another guy, he was devastated. But his emotions proved to be a great motivation for him during the hot two-a-day practices. He was so bummed out and jealous of Sydney's new boyfriend that he threw his heart and soul into practices, taking out all his aggressions on the practice field.

By October, Sydney had broken up with the new guy and was giving Chase big smiles and major hints that she was free again. At an after-game celebration, Chase's resolve to make her wait completely melted when she bounded up and hugged him. A quick kiss turned into a late-night makeout session, and before he knew it, they were right back where they had left off. That first night, he wasn't prepared with condoms. On the exam table, as he contemplated the cluster of bumps on his genitals, he thought back to that hasty decision.

Chase didn't have to wait very long for the doctor. He heard a knock, followed by Dr. Morris's voice asking, "Ready?" She came in and sat on her stool. The nurse, who had followed her in, went over to the corner behind Chase and was busy setting something out on the countertops. Chase knew that it was the policy of this office to have a nurse "chaperone" any time a patient's private parts were examined. He remembered his initial embarrassment during an annual checkup when Dr. Morris taught him how to perform a testicular self-exam for cancer and when she did the dreaded "turn your head and cough" check for a hernia. Over the years, his comfort level had increased to where he barely noticed the nurse, but today he was embarrassed to have anyone other than Dr. Morris around to see this.

"Okay, Chase, so you've got some bumps?," the doctor asked. Suddenly, his mouth went dry, and he couldn't speak. He nodded his head yes. He was relieved that, as usual, she was direct. "When did you first notice them?"

"About three weeks ago," he managed to croak.

"Do they hurt?"

"No." He was grateful for the yes-no question.

"Itch?"

"No."

"But they're getting worse?"

Chase swallowed hard and made eye contact with Dr. Morris. "Um, yeah. There are more of them."

"Have you had sex?," she asked. Now he was really squirming. How many times had she talked to him about using condoms?

"Yes." He knew what was coming next.

"And did you use condoms?"

He couldn't look up any longer. "Mostly," he managed to stammer.

Dr. Morris half smiled and raised her right eyebrow. "'Mostly,' meaning there were times that you had sex that you did not wear a condom?"

"Uh, right," confessed Chase.

"Well, Chase, with skin things, a picture's often worth a thousand words. Let's take a look and see what we're talking about." She put on a pair of gloves and slid out the bottom section of the table so he could fit onto it with his feet extended. "Go ahead and lie back," she said. She lifted the drape and began examining his bumps.

"So, uh, Dr. Morris, do you think it could just be a rash from my jock strap?," he asked hopefully.

"I'm sorry, Chase, but I don't think so. Sit up for a second and let's look at the tops of the bumps. Do you see how wrinkly they look? These are warts."

Warts? His stomach sank. Geez, his worst fears were right. He hadn't realized how much he had been counting on those fears being wrong.

"Okay, Chase, we need to talk about treatment."

Chase was freaking out about having warts. A sexually transmitted infection—gross. They had seen pictures in their health class, but everyone had just laughed and made jokes. It wasn't funny at all now, when it was him with the infection. What was Sydney going to think? Suddenly, it hit him. Sydney. Why was he worried about what she thought? She had probably given the warts to him. She must have slept with that jerk when they broke up last summer.

"Chase? Are you listening?," Dr. Morris asked.

"I'm sorry, Dr. Morris. I was just wondering how I got these. I mean, I know how I got them, but..."

"It's okay. Let's talk about treatment first, and then after you get dressed, I will tell you everything you need to know about warts, including what you need to tell your girlfriend. There are several methods used to treat genital warts. We can use topical acids to burn them, or liquid nitrogen to freeze them. For yours, I think we should use the liquid nitrogen. We can do that right now, in a matter of minutes. You know I'm always honest with you, Chase, so I will tell you that it is going to hurt. It burns pretty badly for about thirty seconds, but then it will just ache. The problem is that after we treat them, the area will blister up, get red, and swell for five to seven days. It will definitely be uncomfortable for you, especially in a jock strap. We could wait until after football season to treat the warts, but they could grow and multiply quite a bit in the next couple of months, so that would not be my recommendation. The smaller they are and the fewer you have, the easier it is to treat them. However, it's your call. I realize this could affect your practice and your game this week. What do you think?"

Chase was still trying to grasp the fact that he had warts—genital warts. He shook his head, trying unsuccessfully to clear his thoughts. "If I do it now, how much do you think it will bug me at practice and during the game? I really just want to get rid of them."

"Well, typically the treatment bothers patients the most during the first few days. It's just hard to say, because wearing football gear might aggravate the area and delay healing a bit. I think you'll be fine, but everyone reacts differently to the freezing, so it's truly hard to predict."

Chase knew there was no way he could delay treatment until December. He felt so gross to have warts down there. There was only one decision. "Let's just treat them now and get it over with. They won't come back, will they?" He looked expectantly at the doctor. Unfortunately, there was no smile now. Dr. Morris looked him right in the eyes.

"Chase, warts are caused by a virus—the human papilloma virus, or HPV for short. There are many different strains, but the thing they all share in common is that we do not yet have a cure for warts. We can treat outbreaks, but we cannot kill the virus. The Gardasil vaccine offers excellent prevention for these warts to those young people who are immunized before they are exposed to HPV, but unfortunately you have not yet had that series of shots."

Chase's mouth dropped open in disbelief. "Are you telling me that if I had agreed to start those shots last year at my physical, I wouldn't have this now? And instead, I'm going to have this the rest of my life?"

"Chase, there is no point in beating yourself up over that decision. A lot of families have been confused about this vaccine, thinking it is only for girls or that it is only to prevent cancer."

"Wait—is that the cancer vaccine my little sister got this year?"

"Yes, exactly. The commercials on TV have really emphasized that this vaccine can prevent cervical cancer in women, and with good reason, since cervical cancer still affects over twelve thousand women each year and kills more than four thousand each year. However, back in 2010, Gardasil was also officially recommended for routine vaccination of boys, partly because it can prevent some less common cancers in males, but also because Gardasil protects everyone against the two strains of HPV that cause ninety percent of genital warts," Dr. Morris explained. "Unfortunately, right now we do not have a cure, so yes, you will carry the virus for the rest of your life. Rest assured, though, just because you have the virus in you does not mean that you will constantly have new crops of warts. Anyway, let's go ahead and treat the ones you've got now, and then after you're dressed, I promise to answer the rest of your questions, okay?"

Chase nodded and lay back on the exam table, closing his eyes.

During this conversation, Debbie had discreetly slipped out of the room, and now she popped back in with a silver canister, which she handed to the doctor. "Chase, this is liquid nitrogen," Dr. Morris said. "I'm going to spray it on each wart until it makes a little frozen ball on top. Then, after they thaw in a few seconds, we repeat that sequence a few times. It will sting and burn while I do this, but it shouldn't take more than five minutes or so to treat all of them. Are you ready?"

Chase felt his heart racing with anxiety as he replied, "Ready as I'll ever be. Go ahead." He watched with a detached fascination as she sprayed each wart. At first the ice ball formed, and he felt nothing, but then came the pain. He gritted his teeth as it began to feel like a bee was stinging him. This would be bad enough for a wart on a finger or a knee, but on his penis? How could this have happened to him?

"Okay, last round. Are you hanging in there?," asked Dr. Morris.

"Yeah. You weren't kidding when you said this would hurt."

Dr. Morris smiled. "You know me, Chase. I always tell the truth. I never tell kids shots don't hurt, so I wouldn't lie about this stinging. Ready?"

"Okay. Tell me when you're done." Chase closed his eyes again and started counting. He figured that if he could focus on counting, she should be finished by the time he got to one hundred. As it turned out, he only had to count to thirty-two.

"Okay, we're done. Debbie is going to put some ointment on the area, and then you can get dressed. I'll come back in a minute and bring you more information about warts." With that, the doctor left the room, and the nurse began smoothing on some ointment.

"This has a little bit of topical anesthetic in it along with the antibiotic, so it should help with the discomfort. Is the stinging going away yet?," asked Debbie.

Chase was just relieved the procedure was finished. "It still burns, but not as bad as when she was spraying that stuff on there."

"Well, it will get better throughout the day. Go ahead and shower normally, cleaning the area with your regular soap and water. The skin is going to blister up and get red before the warts go away. See how it's already swollen?"

Chase looked at his crotch. Everywhere the spray had touched was now bright red and starting to swell. "Man, I sure hope no one notices this in the showers after practice," he thought.

"Give yourself a minute when you sit up before you get dressed," said Debbie. "You might feel a bit light-headed." Then the nurse left the room, and Chase was alone.

He felt tears welling up in his eyes. How could he have warts? The question kept circling around in his brain. Because you had sex without a condom, you idiot, came the answer. What was he going to say to Sydney? He must have gotten the infection from her. Did she know she had warts? He certainly had never seen any on her, not that he'd exactly been looking. "For the rest of your life," the doctor had said. Man, he was only eighteen.

Knock, knock. "Ready?," In came Dr. Morris. Chase was back in his jeans and sitting on the exam table.

"I'm sure you've got a lot of questions for me, Chase. I brought you some handouts on the wart virus for you to take home and read later. Make sure you check out the website on the bottom because it answers a ton of common questions. Right now, though, let's talk about some basics. Genital warts are a sexually transmitted infection, as I'm sure you know. Many people carry the wart virus without realizing that they are infected. Women can actually have warts internally, inside their vaginas, and not be able to see them. Often, the only way women know that they carry the virus is through an abnormal Pap smear, which is a screening test for cervical cancer. Obviously, you need to talk with anyone you've had sex with. Have you had more than one partner?"

"I had sex once a year ago with someone else, but I've only been with my girlfriend, Sydney, in the past six months."

"Well, technically, it's possible that you could have received the virus from either girl, but given the timing, it's more likely that it came from Sydney. Do you happen to know if she has had the Gardasil vaccine?"

"I have no idea. We never talked about it," sighed Chase.

"You'll need to tell her and encourage her to get examined by her doctor," said Dr. Morris. "Anyway, back to you. Please know that even when you don't have any visible warts, you can still pass on the virus. So you absolutely need to use condoms any time that you have sex from now on, and even then, you need to tell your partner that you're a carrier of the virus, since condoms are not foolproof."

"Honestly, right now, the thought of ever having sex with anyone again is the last thing on my mind," said Chase.

Dr. Morris smiled. "I certainly can understand that, but the truth is that you are young, and chances are that you will want to have sex in the future, so I want you to have all the information you need. Do you have any other questions right now?"

Chase thought for a minute. It was hard to digest all this information at once. He glanced at the brochures in his hands. "No, I'm sure these will cover any other questions that I have." All of a sudden, he remembered his mom in the waiting area. What was he going to tell her?

"Wait. I do have a question," he said quickly.

Dr. Morris sat back down. "No problem. What else?"

"Um, my mom is here. Do we have to tell her about this?"

Dr. Morris sighed. "Chase, I recommend that you do tell her. You are eighteen, which means that legally we do not have to tell her anything about your medical care. However, on the bill, under the procedure codes, it's going to say that we treated some warts, so your mom will find out when she gets the bill from the insurance company."

"Can't you just put something else down for the bill?," Chase almost begged.

"No, I'm sorry, I really can't, because that's insurance fraud. That would get me in trouble. It's your decision what you tell her though. It doesn't specify genital warts."

"So I could say that I had a groin pull, but that you also treated a wart somewhere else, like on my leg or something?," he pleaded.

"That would be your choice. But Chase, if your mom asks me a question directly, I won't lie. Now that you're eighteen, I am legally obligated to tell her that I cannot talk to her without your permission, but I won't make anything up to cover, or tell her anything that's not true. Actually, here in California and in most states, since this is a sexually transmittable infection, you have the right to decide about your treatment regardless of your age, without the knowledge or consent of your parents."

Chase felt miserable. He could just see the looks of shock and disappointment and the tears that were sure to come if his mom found out the truth. Not to mention his dad—Chase couldn't even imagine his response. "I understand. You've always treated me right, and I don't want to get you in trouble for my screwup. I... I just don't think I can tell her today, Dr. Morris. I promise to come up with a way to talk to her about this before she hears anything from the insurance company."

Chase stood up and shook the doctor's hand. "Thanks a lot. I'll read this stuff, and I swear I'll be more careful in the future," he said.

"I'm sure you will, Chase. Let's schedule a follow-up appointment in two weeks, to be sure that the warts have completely resolved. They were very small, but most of the time these warts require two or three treatments before we can make them disappear. And feel free to call with any questions that come up that aren't answered in those handouts or on the website."

The two of them stepped out of the room, and Chase began to walk down the hallway.

"Oh, Chase? One more thing." Chase spun around, wondering what she could have forgotten to tell him. Dr. Morris just grinned and added, "Knock 'em dead for the rest of the season."

Chase had to smile. If only everything were as easy as football.

4: Chloe

CHLOE CLOSED HER EYES as she partied on the dance floor, tossing her long, curly black hair to the beat. Aiden's eyes crawled along Chloe's long athletic legs and tight black miniskirt. Even with her sexy red stiletto heels, the top of Chloe's head barely reached his chin. Aiden's lanky six foot six frame was a natural advantage on Tech's cross-country track team, but here on the dance floor he felt like an awkward giant. As the packed crowd swayed and shoved Aiden awkwardly into Chloe yet again, he decided he'd had enough dancing. "Come on." He motioned to Chloe. "Let's take a break and get something to drink."

Aiden grabbed Chloe's hand, and her heart soared as she followed him, looking around the crowded bar to see if any of her friends had spied her holding hands with Aiden. Chloe's first year at Tech had been comfortably filled with dates, but she had been hoping to go out with Aiden since she met him at a tailgate party at the beginning of the year. He literally stood out in a crowd, towering above most of their classmates.

Aiden and Chloe shared the same biology class, along with a couple of hundred other freshmen, but both of them liked to sit in the back row, right by the doors. Chloe thought it was funny how everyone tended to sit in the same spot, as though there were assigned seating in the huge auditorium. That tendency allowed her to get to know the small group of students who sat in her area, including Aiden. Despite Chloe's hopeful flirtations, Aiden had never asked her out, but tonight when they ran into each other at the club, he finally seemed interested. Chloe had actually asked him to dance, but now here he was, gripping her hand and smiling down at her.

"What do you want to drink?," shouted Aiden over the music.

"Diet Coke," Chloe hollered back.

Aiden ordered their drinks and a basket of chips, and then lunged for a nearby table that had just opened up. Chloe happily slid into the chair that Aiden held out.

"Great job snagging a table," she complimented, reaching down to rub her aching feet.

"I hope I'm not the reason your feet hurt," said Aiden sheepishly. "I know I must have stepped on your toes more than once out there."

"No, really, it's just the high heels," laughed Chloe. "I'm far more comfortable in my sneakers, but they didn't quite go with this outfit."

Aiden smiled at his mental image of Chloe in her sexy top and short skirt paired with tennis shoes. "I don't know why not. At least you'd be more comfortable. Anyway, you look great. You should wear this outfit to biology class," he joked.

"Thanks, maybe I will. Are you ready for the test next Friday?," Chloe asked.

"Not yet. Why don't we grab dinner on Thursday, and we can study together afterward?," Aiden asked smoothly.

"Sure, that sounds great." Chloe smiled, as she inwardly jumped up and down. Their conversation flowed easily as they polished off their chips and sodas. Too soon, Aiden's roommate, Isaac, rushed up, grabbing Aiden by the arm. "Come on, Aiden. Sorry to interrupt, but we were supposed to be at Morgan's party an hour ago. I've been looking all over for you." Isaac gave Chloe an apologetic look and added, "Morgan's my girlfriend. She's going to kill me if we're any later."

"Sorry, Chloe, but I really do have to go. I'm the designated driver tonight, and we promised Morgan we were just stopping by here for a few minutes." Aiden stood to go. "We're on for next Thursday though, right?"

"It's a date," Chloe agreed with a smile. She watched the two guys head out of the club, then searched for her friends to share the news. She found Amelia and Kate in the bathroom, touching up their lipstick and hair.

"You did it," squealed Amelia.

"Aiden is so cute," gushed Kate. "I'm so proud of you for asking him to dance. You guys were out there a long time."

"And I saw you over in the corner at a table," added Amelia. "So, tell us everything."

"He actually asked me out!" Chloe recounted her conversation with Aiden, and the girls' chatter continued as Chloe went into a stall. When she wiped herself, she was surprised to see a bit of blood on the toilet paper. "Hey, does anyone have a tampon with them? I can't believe my period just started. It's not due for another week or so," Chloe complained. Unfortunately, her friends had only brought their money, IDs, and phones to the club so they didn't have to hassle with a large purse, and naturally the machine in the bathroom was out of feminine hygiene products.

"Oh well, no big deal. I'm going to head back to the dorm and call it a night," Chloe said as the young women left the bathroom.

"At least you don't have to just dream about Aiden anymore," Amelia said encouragingly. "You can look forward to next week. Kate and I have got to get back out on that dance floor and see if we can meet some decent guys. Wish us luck."

Chloe headed back to her dorm, caught up again in the excitement of her evening. As she showered, she felt a couple of small bumps below her vagina. When she got out and toweled off, there was another spot of blood, so she tried to look in the mirror to figure out where the spotting was coming from. It was an incredibly awkward position, so Chloe couldn't see well enough to be sure, but it looked like the spots of blood were coming from her rectum, not from a period starting early. She got dressed and went to her computer.

"Okay, what the heck do I call this?," Chloe wondered, as she pulled up her favorite search engine. "How about rectal bleeding?" Links to more than a million sites popped up. "Seriously?," she thought to herself, but she began to click on the sites that looked the most official. Chloe read through the descriptions, and because she had no history of abdominal cramps or diarrhea, she assumed she had developed hemorrhoids. "Wow, age eighteen, and I've already got an old lady's problem," Chloe thought. She'd overheard some of her mom's friends complaining about hemorrhoids after having babies. Chloe entered "hemorrhoids" in her search engine, then chose the Mayo Clinic website, figuring that it must be reliable. Mayo's site cautioned that while hemorrhoids are common, if a person has new rectal bleeding, a doctor should determine the cause. Chloe decided she would call for an appointment next week if the spotting continued, then logged off her computer and climbed into bed, not thinking at all about rectal bleeding but happily replaying the evening with Aiden.

Several weeks went by, and Chloe more or less forgot about the whole bleeding episode. No pain or cramps, and she hadn't noticed any new spotting. Nothing could have been further from her mind as she gathered up her dirty clothes and tossed them into her laundry basket. However, as Chloe sorted her colors and whites, she noticed some stains on her underwear from the day before. "Bummer, I thought that had disappeared," she puzzled. Chloe stopped loading the clothes and went to the bathroom to investigate. Sure enough, the spotting was back again today. Since Chloe had finished her period over a week ago, she was pretty sure the bleeding was not from that.

Chloe's thoughts raced: "I guess I didn't notice my underwear last night, since I got changed in the dark." Chloe and Aiden were becoming regular night owls, so Chloe had started getting ready for bed with the light off so she wouldn't wake her roommate when she came in from a late date. Chloe's thoughts drifted back to last night. "I can't believe how we love all the same things—Asian food, mountain biking, and watching old movies. It's almost too good to be true." She quickly knocked on wood, warding off any jinx her thoughts may have triggered. "Okay, Chloe, focus," she sternly told herself and grabbed her phone to look up the number for the health center.

Just a few hours later, Chloe was on an exam table, nervously sitting half naked with a sheet draped over her legs. The nurse, Maureen, was setting out scary-looking equipment on a nearby tray table. "What's that?," Chloe asked apprehensively.

"This is a pelvic speculum, and this smaller one is an anoscope," Maureen replied matter-of-factly. "Haven't you had a pelvic exam before?"

"No, I most certainly have not," exclaimed Chloe. "Does the doctor have to put that thing inside me? It looks huge."

"Really, it's not that bad," reassured Maureen. "You'll feel some pressure, but not pain."

"But I'm a virgin," protested Chloe. "I mean, I use tampons, of course, but that thing is way bigger than a tampon."

"Don't worry, Dr. Lopez is really gentle. I'll be sure to tell him that this will be your first pelvic exam. If you just have hemorrhoids, he might be able to see what's going on without even using any of this. Please try to relax, and he and I will be back in the room in a minute."

Chloe swallowed hard as the nurse whisked out of the room and closed the door. She shifted back and forth on the table, way too nervous to just relax, as Maureen had suggested. Her eyes were drawn to the tray table, focusing on the two instruments and the numerous swabs that had been set out. "All this for a little spotting," thought Chloe. "Maybe I overreacted, and I really don't need any of this." She was seriously thinking about getting dressed and leaving, when Maureen and the doctor came in.

Dr. Lopez had dark, thick hair and a mustache. He was short and stocky, with a muscular chest and arms. His light blue button-down shirt was neatly pressed, matching his starched white coat. "Hi, I'm

Dr. Lopez," he greeted Chloe, extending his hand. "So I understand that you've noticed some spotting on your underwear, is that right?"

"Yes, just a couple of times," answered Chloe.

"When did you first notice it?"

"About a month ago, on a Friday night. At first I thought I was going to start my period, but then by the next day, the spotting was gone," said Chloe. "I didn't notice any again until today."

"And now you think it's coming from your rectum?," inquired Dr. Lopez.

"I think so. Do people my age get hemorrhoids?"

"Actually, hemorrhoids are fairly common in college students, because their diet is often pretty low in fiber. Are you a burger and pizza girl, or do you try to maintain a healthy diet?," asked Dr. Lopez.

"I think I eat far better than the average college student," Chloe bragged. "I grew up always eating plenty of fruits and vegetables, so I have a banana with breakfast most days, and I always snack on apples and grapes. My friends actually tease me because I also love those high-fiber snack bars."

"Have you had any diarrhea or constipation lately?," he asked.

"Not that I've noticed," Chloe replied.

Dr. Lopez made some notes in Chloe's chart and then looked up. "I see that you have regular periods, and that you have not been sexually active yet. Is that correct?"

Chloe blushed. "That's right."

"Okay, then. Please lie back so we can make sure you don't have any extra lumps or bumps anywhere, and we'll see what seems to be causing this spotting."

Chloe began to lie back on the table as Maureen stepped over and pulled out the stirrups. "Oh, speaking of bumps, last month I thought I felt some small ones around my bottom when I saw that spotting, but I couldn't see anything with a mirror."

Dr. Lopez and Maureen exchanged a look, which didn't escape notice by Chloe. Casually, Dr. Lopez continued his questions. "What kind of bumps? Could you see or feel how big they were?"

"They were small, maybe pea-sized. Does that sound like a hemorrhoid?," she asked hopefully. She felt sweat break out on her palms.

"Just go ahead and lie back, and we'll take a look," he said.

Chloe followed his directions, trying to keep her knees apart as Maureen gently directed her. She watched Dr. Lopez put on his gloves and begin to examine her. Almost immediately, he reported, "Okay, I see the problem here. I need to use this small scope to look inside though. Just try and relax, and I'll be done in a minute."

Before she knew it, Chloe felt the instrument enter her rectum. She thought she might die from embarrassment or fear, but the procedure was done fairly quickly. Or so she thought.

"Now I need to do the pelvic exam," Dr. Lopez revealed.

"What?" Chloe sat halfway up, rising up on her elbows, but with her feet still in the stirrups. "Do you remember that I haven't had sex yet?," she protested.

"Yes, Chloe, I do remember that. Unfortunately, it looks like those bumps that you felt are not hemorrhoids, but actually anal warts, which is a sexually transmitted infection. I need to look in your vagina to make sure that you don't have any warts inside," Dr. Lopez said.

Chloe was incredulous. She thought to herself, "Anal warts? How disgusting can you get?" But she didn't say anything; she simply fell back and endured the pelvic exam.

"Okay, you can sit up now. We went ahead and checked you for other STIs. The only warts that I saw in the exam were the few near your anus, one of which was bleeding slightly. I assume that's what's causing your spotting," the doctor said.

"Warts? Are you sure it's warts down there?," Chloe asked.

"Yes, Chloe. We see these pretty frequently. Typically, it's from anal sex. Do you think that might be how you got yours?," he asked gently.

Tears filled Chloe's eyes. "I swear," she sobbed. "I didn't think you could catch anything from doing that. It's not real sex! And I've only done it a few times."

The doctor looked uncomfortable, but Maureen smiled and touched Chloe's knee sympathetically. Chloe rushed through the rest of her explanation. "I... I realize this probably sounds stupid or silly to you, but I planned to save real sex for when I am married, or at least engaged. It's against my religion." Chloe broke down and started crying.

"I'm sorry," said Dr. Lopez, "and you are absolutely not alone in thinking that 'real sex'—meaning vaginal intercourse—is the only way to catch an STI. The truth is, however, that you can get virtually every sexually transmittable infection via either anal sex or even 'just' oral sex. Many young people choosing 'abstinence' for religious reasons are ending up with STIs because they don't realize these facts."

Sympathetically, the doctor continued, "At any rate, if you'd like me to start treating the warts today, I'll need you to lie back down. It's going to sting a bit. Maureen, can you grab the liquid nitrogen from the cabinet?"

"*Start* treating them? How long does it take?," Chloe asked.

"I don't know yet how many times you'll need. We'll have to see you back in two weeks, and likely repeat the treatment. Usually, it takes several visits to get rid of a crop of these warts. Luckily, I didn't see any inside your rectum or your vagina. That would have been a much bigger deal. We send those to the specialists to treat."

"What are you going to use on me today?," Chloe asked. Dr. Lopez held up the bottle Maureen had just handed him and showed it to Chloe. "I prefer treating warts like yours with liquid nitrogen. TCA, which is an acid, can also be used, but it can be a little tough on the anal area. There is another milder medicine that patients can use at home, but I find it is not as successful. Besides, where your warts are, they're pretty hard for you to see, so I think you'll do much better if we just treat you here."

"As long as you get rid of them, I'm with you," sighed Chloe, lying back once again and finding the stirrups with her feet.

Dr. Lopez began to apply the liquid nitrogen, and Chloe realized she was biting her lip to keep from crying. The sharp burning pain made it nearly impossible to keep her legs open as the doctor treated the warts. "How many are there?," Chloe managed to squeak out between applications.

"Looks like there are just four," replied Dr. Lopez. "Okay, I'm finished." He walked around the side of the exam table so he could look directly at Chloe. "Please schedule an appointment for two weeks from now, and we'll repeat this treatment again. We hope that these warts will completely disappear within two to three months."

"Months?"

"Yes, months. But Chloe, just because these warts clear up, it doesn't mean the virus is gone. Also, about twenty-five percent of people with newly diagnosed anal warts have a recurrence within the first three months after treatment."

Chloe rose up on her elbows again, challenging: "What? I thought you said this treatment would make them go away."

"All warts are caused by a virus, Chloe, and we don't yet have a cure for the virus. Maureen will get you a handout that explains all this. The virus is called HPV, which stands for the human papilloma virus. There are lots of different strains of HPV. Types six and eleven cause the vast majority of genital warts, roughly ninety percent, but luckily, they don't appear to cause cancer. It is possible, though less likely, for genital or anal warts to be caused by other strains of HPV that can cause vulvar, anal, or penile cancer. HPV types sixteen and eighteen have the strongest link to cervical cancer but rarely cause visible warts like you have."

Chloe lay back down and closed her eyes, confused and speechless. Dr. Lopez continued, "Also, I recommend that you get the first dose of the Gardasil vaccine today. Although we know you have at least one type of HPV causing your warts, Gardasil works against all four HPV types that I mentioned—types six and eleven, which cause genital warts, and types sixteen and eighteen, which cause seventy percent of all cervical cancers. The vaccine is a series of three injections that you receive over six months. It's believed that the majority of sexually active adults harbor the HPV infection, although most don't know it because they don't have symptoms. In fact, the Centers for Disease Control say that nearly eighty million Americans at any given time have active HPV, and roughly seventy-five percent of Americans aged fifteen to forty-nine years old have been infected at some point. Obviously, this makes HPV by far the most common STI in the United States. Chances are that you don't yet have the types of HPV that cause cervical cancer, and the vaccine would help you avoid getting it."

"So you're telling me that I'm stuck with this virus forever, even if we make the warts go away, and even if I get the vaccine. Is that right?," Chloe asked.

"Yes. However, as long as we treat outbreaks and screen you regularly, my hope is that it won't bother you that much," replied Dr. Lopez. "When you decide to be sexually active in the future, you should let your partner know that you have the virus. We will hope that your partner will already be vaccinated against HPV, which would dramatically lower any risk of transmission. Additionally, we know that condoms can significantly reduce the risk for HPV-related diseases, meaning both warts and cancer. Condoms are not by any means foolproof though, because the virus can be present on areas that condoms don't cover, like the scrotum or anus in guys, or the vulva or anus in girls. Does that make sense?"

Chloe nodded, trying to process everything the doctor had said and doing her best to ignore the searing pain in her bottom.

"Okay, then, I'll see you in a couple of weeks," Dr. Lopez said as he left the room.

Maureen put away her supplies and turned back to Chloe, peeking under her drape to check the warts. "All right, honey, you can get up now. I put a two-pack of ibuprofen on the counter for you to help with the discomfort, right next to the HPV handout. I'll give you a few minutes to get dressed, and then I'll come back with your first dose of Gardasil, assuming you want to get it."

"Absolutely," said Chloe. "I still can't believe I've got *any* kind of HPV. If that shot will help protect me from getting other ones, I'm all for it." Chloe shook her head incredulously. "Is it true that if I had gotten the vaccine a few years ago, I wouldn't be sitting here right now?"

"Honestly, most likely not, but please don't beat yourself up about it, Chloe," reassured Maureen. "Unfortunately, only about a third of eligible girls and even fewer boys have completed their HPV vaccine series so far. Gardasil was approved by the FDA all the way back in June 2006 (for girls) and in 2009 (for boys), and clinicians *should* have been including HPV vaccination as part of routine immunizations for both boys and girls since 2011. However, many families *and sometimes even their clinicians* have skipped this series of shots. Sometimes people mistakenly believe the HPV vaccine is not necessary in their socioeconomic group, or they have chosen for other reasons not to get this immunization."

"That's so true! I know my parents told our doctor that I wasn't the 'type of young lady' who would need such a vaccine," sighed Chloe. "But here I am..."

Chloe got dressed, received her vaccine, and scheduled her follow-up appointment. She carefully walked across campus, trying not to aggravate her sore spots, oblivious to the sunshine and crisp weather. "Anal warts. I have anal warts. Oh my gosh, how did I let this happen?" The thoughts were stuck in her head, playing over and over with every painful step toward her dorm. "Who gave me HPV? I've only been with a few guys. Could it have been Adam? He turned out to be such a player. Or maybe Carter? Did he know he had HPV? Did he lie to me? Who gave me these warts? How could I end up with anal warts?" And she was back in the painful loop again. As Chloe opened the door to her dorm, her cell phone chirped. The text was from Aiden. "Study break? Let's bike over to Double Dips for ice cream."

Tears overflowing, Chloe could only think sarcastically, "Oh yeah, great idea. Sure, sitting on a bike seat with my rear end on fire sounds absolutely wonderful right now." But she knew her anger wasn't directed at Aiden. The reality of her infection was sinking in. What would she tell Aiden? *Would* she tell him? What would she think if it were the other way around, and Aiden told her that he had anal warts? Had Aiden gotten his HPV shots yet? It was just too much to absorb right now. Chloe typed back, "I wish! Too much homework. Maybe next time..."

"One step at a time," she thought, taking a deep breath. "I'll deal with this and figure it out. Me and eighty million other Americans."

facts

Human Papilloma Virus (HPV) Fact Sheet

What is it?

- HPV is a group of over 100 viral subtypes, more than 30 of which are transmitted sexually.

- Types 16 and 18 cause 70% of cervical cancers.

- Types 6 and 11 cause 90% of genital warts.

- Other types cause the "common" warts on hands or feet.

How common is it?

- As of 2014 the CDC estimated that 79 million people in the United States (nearly 25% of the population) are actively infected at any given time with sexually transmitted HPV, *although the vast majority of these people do not know they are infected.* This virus is so prevalent that it is believed that most sexually active men and women will acquire some type of HPV in their lifetime.

- 14 million Americans are newly infected each year.
- Over 1 million people have visible genital warts at any given time in the United States.
- HPV is the most common sexually transmitted infection in the United States.

How do you get it?

- Through skin-to-skin contact with an infected partner, with the thin skin of the genitals being most easily infected. (HPV does not live in blood, semen, or vaginal secretions.)
- Through oral, vaginal, or anal sex.
- Less commonly, HPV genital wart types can be passed to a baby during vaginal childbirth, causing serious problems with warts in the infant's larynx, eyes, or genitals.

Where on your body do you get it?

- In women, genital warts can occur on the labia, in the vagina, on the cervix, anywhere in the anal or genital area, and on the abdomen or thighs.
- In men, genital warts can occur in the urethral opening, on the penis, scrotum, or anus, and on the abdomen or thighs.

How do I know if I have it?

- Most people are asymptomatic, so women are often diagnosed through routine cervical cancer screening tests: the Pap test and specific HPV DNA tests.
- There are no HPV screening tests for males (other than as part of a research study).
- A small percentage of people infected with HPV grow genital warts, which are typically painless.
- Warts in the opening of the urethra can cause blood in the urine.
- Warts can itch or bleed, though most do not.
- Coating the genitals with vinegar can make warts turn white, making them easier to see; however, some benign skin conditions may also turn white.

What does it look like?

- Normal anatomy or flesh-colored, flat or raised wrinkled bumps, singly or in groups.

What does it feel like?

- Most people are unaware that they have HPV.
- 20% of people with genital warts experience itching.

How long does it last?

- The vast majority of HPV infections clinically resolve within a few years. However, those people who end up with persistent infections have an increased risk for HPV-related cancers.

- 20% of genital warts resolve without treatment (meaning, the visible warts disappear, but the infection remains).

- 25% of genital warts recur in the first three months after treatment.

Can it be cured?

- No. Treatments can remove visible warts, but recurrence is common, and potential infectivity is permanent.

- Infectivity is thought to be greater when there are untreated, visible warts.

Can you be reinfected?

- No, not with the same strain of HPV.

- Rarely, people autoinoculate (meaning, they transmit HPV from their genitals to another location on their own body).

What is the treatment?

- Multiple treatments exist, and type of treatment depends on location, number, and size of warts, as well as physician and patient preference.

Treatments performed by providers:

- Cryotherapy: freezing with liquid nitrogen; treatments repeated every one to two weeks until warts have resolved.

- TCA (trichloroacetic acid) or BCA (bichloroacetic acid): acids that chemically burn the warts; they dry to a white crust; treatments repeated every one to two weeks until warts are resolved.

- Podophyllin: applied to wart and often washed off 1–4 hours later; not indicated for pregnant women.

- Laser: usually for extensive warts, intraurethral warts, or those resistant to other therapy.
- Surgery: treatment is usually complete in one visit; higher risk of scarring.

Treatments applied by patients (should be discussed with physician first):

- Podofilox: applied with swab twice daily for 3 days, then 4 days without treatment; treatment may be repeated up to 4 cycles. Ideally, physician should perform first application to confirm warts and safety of this method.
- Imiquimod: applied at bedtime 3 nights per week for up to 16 weeks; washed off 6–10 hours later.

How about alternative therapies?

- Interferon injections directly into wart lesions are not recommended as a primary treatment due to high incidence of side effects and necessity of multiple treatments.
- No herbal or home remedies are proven to eliminate HPV.
- Swabbing of the genital area with vinegar may help patients and partners identify new warts.

Are there long-term consequences of HPV?

- Types 16 and 18 cause 70% of cervical cancers.
- There are 14 strains of HPV (16, 18, 31, 33, 35, 39, 45, 51, 52, 56, 58, 59, 66, 68) that are considered high risk because of their link with cervical, vaginal, anal, and other squamous cell cancers.

They can be occasionally found in genital warts, although 90% of genital warts are caused by types 6 and 11, which are not precancerous.

When are you contagious?

- Any time you are infected with HPV, regardless of symptoms.
- Even while using a condom. Latex male condoms can reduce but not eliminate transmission of HPV, since HPV is present on genital surfaces not covered with a condom.

How do I avoid getting HPV?

- Completely abstaining from oral, vaginal, and anal sex, as well as direct skin-to-skin genital contact, is the only way to be 100% sure of avoiding contracting HPV.
- Gardasil vaccine offers protection against HPV types 6 and 11, which cause 90% of genital warts, and types 16 and 18, which cause 70% of cervical cancers.
- Gardasil-9 was FDA approved in December 2014 and provides additional protection against 5 more types of HPV (31, 33, 45, 52, 58), which cause another 20% of cervical cancers.
- Condoms can significantly decrease but not eliminate transmission of HPV.

Who should get the HPV vaccine?

- HPV vaccination is recommended for all children as part of routine immunizations at age 11 or 12. If missed at that age, then catch-up vaccination is suggested for females up to age 26 and males up to age 21. Additionally, men who have sex with men are recommended to get this vaccine up through age 26.

Is the HPV vaccine effective?

- Studies have shown the HPV vaccines to be incredibly effective, with efficacy rates better than 95% in preventing genital warts and cervical precancers and cancers.
- From 2006, when HPV vaccines began to be recommended as part of the routine immunization schedule, to 2010, the number of HPV infections in teenage girls in the United States fell by 56%.
- In Australia there is widespread, free HPV immunization for school-age girls, and studies there show the additional benefit of "herd immunity," noting a dramatic decrease of genital warts in both sexes. Even though boys had not received the HPV vaccine series themselves, their chances of acquiring the infection decreased because fewer girls had HPV infections.

Is the HPV vaccine safe?

- Yes. As of 2014, over 170 million doses have been administered worldwide, including over 67 million doses in the United States, and there are no serious adverse reactions consistently related to the vaccine.
- Due to a slightly increased incidence of fainting with this vaccine, the CDC and the FDA suggest remaining seated (or lying down) for 15 minutes immediately after receiving each dose.

If I have HPV, how do I avoid giving it to my partner?

- Your partner should be immunized with the Gardasil vaccine for protection against acquiring HPV types 6, 11, 16, and 18.
- Condom use is recommended and significantly reduces (although it cannot eliminate) transmission of HPV.

- Direct skin-to-skin contact involving the genital area of an infected person can transmit HPV, so abstain from "dry humping" (genital contact without vaginal or anal penetration) as well as intercourse.

Does HPV transmission occur in homosexual partners?

- HPV is transmitted through skin-to-skin contact with an infected partner, regardless of gender.
- HPV transmission does occur in women who have sex with women, although documentation is limited (because many studies include women who have bisexual as well as homosexual contacts).
- HPV can be contracted through receiving anal intercourse.

Frequently Asked Questions

➤ **How common is HPV?**
Extremely common. More than 79 million Americans are infected with this virus.

➤ **Will my genital warts turn into cancer?**
Although the risk is not zero, it's very unlikely. Typically the strains that cause genital warts do not cause cancers.

➤ **If I just developed warts, did my current partner cheat on me?**
Not necessarily. The HPV virus can be dormant for weeks, months, years, or even a lifetime. It is not known what triggers an outbreak of warts, although stress and immune status are thought to play a role. Your current partner or a former partner may be one of the many Americans with silent, and therefore undiagnosed, HPV.

➤ **To catch HPV, do you have to have sex with multiple partners?**

No. Although your risk of any STI increases with the number of partners you have had, HPV is so common that you can easily contract it from even your first partner (unless neither of you has had any prior genital contact).

➤ **If I get the Gardasil vaccine, will I still need to use condoms?**
Yes. Gardasil only works against HPV. The injection offers no protection from any other sexually transmitted infection.

➤ **Can my male partner be tested for HPV?**
There are no tests currently available outside of research settings to screen men for HPV.

Additional Information

American College of Obstetricians and Gynecologists
PO Box 70620
Washington, DC 20024-9998
1-800-673-8444
www.acog.org/departments/dept_notice.cfm?recno=7&bulletin=3097

American Sexual Health Association
PO Box 13827
Research Triangle Park, NC 27709
919-361-8400
www.ashasexualhealth.org/

Centers for Disease Control and Prevention
1600 Clifton Road
Atlanta, GA 30329-4027
1-800-CDC-INFO (1-800-232-4636), 1-888-232-6348 (TTY)
www.cdc.gov/std/hpv/default.htm

HPV Vaccine—Questions and Answers
www.cdc.gov/vaccines/vpd-vac/hpv/vac-faqs.htm

MedlinePlus
US National Library of Medicine
8600 Rockville Pike
Bethesda, MD 20894
1-888-FIND-NLM (1-888-346-3656) or 301-594-5983
www.nlm.nih.gov/medlineplus/hpv.html

National Cancer Institute
9609 Medical Center Drive
Bethesda, MD 20892-9760
1-800-4-CANCER (1-800-422-6237)
www.cancer.gov/cancertopics/factsheet/Risk/HPV

CERVICAL CANCER

5: Rachel

RACHEL HAD BEEN SITTING in the waiting room of the gynecologist for over an hour. As a grade-school art teacher, it was extremely difficult to get time off to go to the doctor, and if she didn't get done soon, she was afraid she wouldn't make it back to teach her afternoon classes. The nurse had come out a while ago to tell everyone that Dr. Butler had been called away to an emergency delivery and asked if anyone wanted to reschedule. Rachel had been somewhat amazed that most of the women declined and went right back to reading various parenting magazines.

Rachel looked around at the obviously pregnant women and wondered when it would be her turn to have a child. Rachel was thirty years old and had been married just over three years. Her husband, Jack, was a civil engineer. He was a compulsively organized, predictable kind of guy. Rachel was much more of a free spirit. They were the ultimate "opposites attract" couple, but their extremes complemented one another beautifully. Jack did all the finances, from paying bills to investments. Rachel was in charge of their social life, cooking, and home decor. She loved to host elaborate, themed wine tastings and holiday parties. They both loved kids and talked about raising three or four of their own. Rachel wasn't desperate to start trying to conceive, but as more of her friends had babies and since she was now officially out of her twenties, Rachel was happy that she and Jack had decided to stop using birth control and let nature take its course this year.

At Jack's insistence, Rachel had gone to see her family physician to get a full physical and "clearance," as he put it, that she was in optimal health and ready to conceive. Rachel had laughed at his concern, telling him that nothing could be wrong with her since she had become a vegetarian and avid yoga practitioner a couple of years ago. Indeed, everything turned out great, except for Rachel's Pap test.

Rachel knew that a Pap test is a screening exam for cervical cancer, but she had never really thought much more about it beyond that fact. She knew her cervix was the bottom part of her womb that opened into her vagina. The nurse who called with her results said that Rachel's Pap test showed some abnormal cells on her cervix that needed further testing. Rachel was not particularly concerned, especially because she recalled that during college she had a couple of Pap tests that were "mildly abnormal," but repeated Pap tests always went back to normal. Besides, she vaguely remembered that the last time she had a physical, the doctor had told her that recommendations for Pap tests had completely changed in 2012, and women did not need to be tested as often as had been previously recommended. But Rachel's primary doctor was now concerned enough to refer her to the gynecologist for further testing, which is why Rachel was here today. Apparently, she was in for a "pretty uncomfortable" experience that included "biopsies" of her cervix, which sounded a bit intimidating. She had taken three ibuprofen tablets before leaving work, as the office had instructed. Rachel didn't want to reschedule an appointment that she had been somewhat dreading and had rearranged her life for.

Finally, about an hour and a half later than her scheduled appointment time, she was brought back into an exam room. The medical assistant, Shelly, took all her vital signs and gave her a patient gown. Shelly sat down at the computer and pulled up Rachel's records. She quickly reassured Rachel that she had electronic copies of Rachel's Pap report, and then began to ask questions about Rachel's gynecological history.

"So, how old were you when your periods started?," Shelly inquired.

"Gosh, I don't know. I think seventh grade—like twelve years old?," Rachel responded.

"Sounds right," Shelly agreed. "And are your periods regular?"

"Yes, but I've been on the pill for a lot of years," said Rachel.

Shelly continued, "Any spotting or bleeding between periods?"

"No, not really," Rachel replied.

"Any spotting after sex?"

"Yes, sometimes that happens, but it's not consistent, and it doesn't hurt or anything," Rachel mused. "Honestly, I couldn't tell you the last time it happened, because I don't pay much attention to it. I thought that happened to everyone.... Is that a bad sign?"

"Well, bleeding after intercourse is not normal, and definitely something you want to check out with your doctor, which is exactly what we are doing today," Shelly answered, making notes on the computer. "Have you ever been pregnant?"

"No, but we're planning to start trying this year."

"Great. Maybe you'll be back soon as an obstetrical patient," Shelly added enthusiastically. "Okay, back to my form. Are you now, or have you ever been, a smoker?"

"Oh, in college I used to smoke socially, but I haven't had a cigarette in years now," replied Rachel.

"Good for you," approved Shelly. "How many total sexual partners have you had? One to five, six to ten, or greater than ten?"

Rachel blushed at this question. She had always been very comfortable with her sexuality, but counting up her encounters felt awkward. She thought about it for a moment, then opted to round down a touch and said, "In the six range."

"Any history of sexually transmitted infections?," Shelly asked.

Rachel was more prepared for this question. "Yes. In college I was treated for chlamydia once."

"Anything else?"

"No, not that I can think of," Rachel replied.

"What about the human papilloma virus?," Shelly asked.

"The what?," asked Rachel.

"HPV, the wart virus. Of course, that's what you've got now, but I was trying to find out if this was the first time it had showed up on your Pap test," Shelly said apologetically.

"Really?," said Rachel. "Actually, they just told me my Pap test was abnormal. I didn't realize it was from a wart virus. That's weird, because I don't think I have any warts."

Shelly reassured Rachel that the majority of the patients they saw with abnormal changes from this virus did not have any associated warts. "The problem is that in addition to the changes on the Pap, you also tested positive for the types of HPV that are high risk for causing cervical cancer. That's why we brought you in to take a look and do a few biopsies to see how best to treat you," explained Shelly.

"Wait, are you saying I could have cancer? Or that I have a wart virus? I'm confused," said Rachel.

Shelly elaborated, "All we know right now is that you have this virus, HPV. And yes, HPV can cause cancer. However, we'll need the results from the biopsies that the doctor will take today to tell us exactly how much, if any, precancerous change you actually have."

"Could it be cancer already?," worried Rachel.

"It's very unlikely in your case, because your Pap test was only mildly abnormal," answered Shelly.

Rachel nodded, but now her heart was racing. She had known that a Pap was a test for cervical cancer, but everyone had seemed so calm about her abnormal test, it hadn't really clicked with her that there could be a serious problem. "But we'll know for sure once the doctor looks at the biopsies? Will that be today?"

"Yes, that should tell us, but we won't know today. It's a pathologist who looks at the biopsies, and it takes a few days to get the results. We'll certainly call you as soon as we hear."

"A few days to worry about whether or not I've got cancer. Great," thought Rachel. She decided she'd better focus on the moment and what to expect from the upcoming procedure.

"Now I'm pretty nervous. Do you knock me out or something? I'm kind of wimpy about pain."

Shelly smiled, "Oh, no. It's like a regular Pap test, but with a pain that feels like a hard menstrual cramp for most people. Did you take some ibuprofen this morning?"

"Yes."

"That's all you'll need. Dr. Butler ought to be here pretty soon, and she'll answer any more questions you might have."

Shelly then went over the consent form for the colposcopy and biopsies and handed it to Rachel to sign. "The doctor is back now, and you're her first patient," said Shelly, "so she should be here any minute."

"Don't worry. I've waited this long, so I'm not going anywhere," Rachel replied.

Dr. Butler popped in the door a few minutes later, with Shelly following behind her. "Hi, I'm Dr. Butler," she said. "Sorry I'm running so far behind, but I was called out for a delivery. Anyway, I'm here now, so let's get started. I'm sure you're anxious to get this over with."

"Definitely," replied Rachel.

"I see you had an abnormal Pap test, and we found cells that can cause cervical cancer, so you're here for further testing. Did Shelly go over everything with you?"

"Pretty much," Rachel shrugged tensely.

"Good. Go ahead and lie back and scoot down," said the doctor.

Rachel did as the doctor instructed, and the next five minutes or so passed in a blur as Rachel used her meditation skills to try to relax to minimize the discomfort. Rachel thought it hurt way more than a menstrual cramp, but she didn't say anything.

"Okay, we're finished. It will take a few days to get the results back from the pathologist, and Shelly will call you then. Meanwhile, let me give you my speech about HPV, okay?"

Rachel was sitting up now, uncomfortable but relieved the procedure was over, and ready to focus on what the doctor was telling her. "Fire away," she said.

"HPV, the human papilloma virus, is extremely common. They estimate that an American's lifetime risk of acquiring it is nearly seventy-five percent. Risk factors for getting it are multiple sexual partners or sex with one high-risk partner, smoking, and a history of having other STIs. There is debate about whether oral contraceptive pills increase or decrease the risk. There are many types of HPV, but only a few are responsible for causing cervical cancer. Another couple of types cause most genital warts. You are here because your Pap test and a DNA test showed that you have the type of HPV that is high risk for causing cancer, so we needed to get some tissue samples to make sure that you don't already have cancerous changes."

"Did it look like cancer to you?," interjected Rachel.

"Your cervix did bleed rather easily, which we call 'friable,' but otherwise, to the naked eye, everything looks normal. The whole point, though, is to find any precancerous or even cancerous cells as early as possible, before it gets to the point where it would be visible on a pelvic exam. If we find any of those cells on your biopsies, then we will need to do another procedure to get rid of those cells and try to prevent any progression toward cancer. Are you with me so far?," she asked.

"Yes," said Rachel. "So I definitely have this wart virus, specifically the kind that wants to cause cancer, not warts, but we don't know yet if it has caused any cancer changes?"

"Exactly," said Dr. Butler.

"And will this affect me getting pregnant?," asked Rachel.

"Not the procedure you've just finished. It would depend on what extra procedures you might need if the biopsies show any cancerous changes," said Dr. Butler.

"So there's no antibiotic to fix this?," asked Rachel.

"Not yet. However, you've probably seen ads for the HPV vaccine, Gardasil. When young girls get this vaccine before they are ever sexually active, this immunization is amazingly effective at preventing HPV-related infection. We're truly optimistic that this vaccine will eliminate cervical cancer. The first generation of HPV vaccines protects against HPV types sixteen and eighteen, which cause seventy percent of cervical cancer. Additionally, Gardasil also protects against genital warts, because it includes the HPV types that cause ninety percent of genital warts—types six and eleven. In 2015, a second generation of HPV vaccine, called Gardasil-9, was FDA approved. It protects against the same four strains that the original HPV vaccine does, but adds in five more cancer-causing strains. Prevention will be our best tool to fight cervical cancer because, unfortunately, there are no antiviral medicines that work against HPV yet," admitted the doctor.

"And what about my husband? Does he need to be tested or treated?," Rachel wondered.

"The only way we're aware that a man has HPV is when he develops genital warts. If you remember what I said earlier, the strain that we know you have can cause cancer, but is highly unlikely to cause warts. So, while we know your husband has been exposed and is most likely infected, we don't yet have any way to detect or treat this strain of virus in him."

"So basically, we just wait to see my results and hope I don't need any further treatment?," said Rachel.

"Yes. We will call you next week and let you know," said Dr. Butler.

"And if it is cancerous? Can you tell me what to expect then?," said Rachel.

"It would depend on the pathology report. Often, we can treat patients with a quick procedure here in the office, using chemicals or liquid nitrogen to destroy the tissue. We also have surgical options, using lasers or loops to remove the tissue. Of course, you would be sedated for those procedures," replied Dr. Butler.

"Are all cervical cancers caused by HPV?," asked Rachel.

"We think so. It's amazing to think that an STI causes cancer, isn't it?," answered the doctor.

"Wait—you consider this an STI even when there are no warts?"

"Definitely. STI simply means that you caught this through sex, and that is how this infection is transmitted."

Rachel let that sink in for a moment and then asked, "How often does the virus actually cause cancer? Does anyone die of cervical cancer anymore?"

"Sadly, yes. Cervical cancer is the second most common cancer in women worldwide, but it doesn't get as much press as breast cancer, even though cervical cancer is preventable. Most years there are approximately twelve thousand women diagnosed with cervical cancer in the United States, and unfortunately there are still about four thousand deaths per year from this cancer," said Dr. Butler. "We've only had one patient in our practice die from it, but that was one too many. I'm not telling you this to scare you, but to emphasize the seriousness of the effects of HPV. With our improving detection of early cellular changes and our better ability to detect the high-risk HPV strains, we are able to cure the vast majority of the cancers that we find."

That certainly put a more intense slant on the whole thing. Rachel made a mental note to thank her diligent husband for pushing her to get that physical. "Well, you've certainly got my attention. I truly had no idea this could be that serious. I guess I'll talk to you ladies next week, then," she said, and thanked both the doctor and her medical assistant. Rachel got dressed and checked out.

As she walked through the waiting room, she looked at the pregnant women with new appreciation. Rachel realized that things she had taken for granted even an hour ago now meant more to her. She looked forward to the time when, rather than dreading a procedure to treat the wart virus, she would be sitting in this room excited to hear her baby's heartbeat. Rachel hoped and prayed she hadn't lost that chance already.

facts

Cervical Cancer Fact Sheet

What is it?

- Cervical cancer is a disease of uncontrolled growth of abnormal cells of the cervix, which is the lower part, or opening, of the uterus.

- Human papilloma virus types 16 and 18 cause 70% of cervical cancers.

- HPV types 16, 18, 31, 33, 45, 52, and 58 are considered the high-risk HPV types because of their link with cervical, vaginal, anal, and other squamous cell cancers.

- 5%–30% of infections will include more than one type of HPV.

How common is it?

- The American Cancer Society estimates that 12,900 women in the United States will be diagnosed with invasive cervical cancer in 2015.
- There will be roughly 4,100 deaths in the United States from cervical cancer in 2015.
- Keep in mind that, although the majority (50%–75%) of sexually active adults in the United States will at some point acquire HPV, only a small percentage will develop cervical cancer.
- Studies have shown that the majority of women who are diagnosed with cervical cancer have not had a Pap test in more than 5 years, if ever.

How do you get it?

- Skin-to-skin contact or intercourse with an infected partner carrying the human papilloma virus.

Where on your body do you get it?

- Cervical cancer starts on the cervix but can extend to include the vaginal wall, uterus, rectum, bladder, lymph nodes, lungs, liver, or other sites.

How do I know if I have it?

- Early on, most infections are asymptomatic and may only be diagnosed during a routine checkup.
- Pap tests detect the types of HPV that cause cervical cancer.
- Not all abnormal Pap tests are precancerous or cancerous; your healthcare professional can explain what your abnormal Pap test

means.

What does it look like?

- Normal anatomy, or red, inflamed cervix. A growth may be visible at later stages.

What does it feel like?

- Most people are unaware they have cervical cancer because at early stages, there are usually no symptoms.
- In more advanced disease, women may notice abnormal vaginal bleeding, including bleeding or spotting between periods, after intercourse, or after menopause and/or menstrual periods that are longer or heavier than normal.
- Increased vaginal discharge, pelvic pain, and dyspareunia (pain with intercourse) can be present in advanced disease.
- Bleeding after intercourse—1 in 220 women with this symptom have invasive cervical cancer.

What is a Pap smear or Pap test?

- A Pap test is a screening exam for cervical cancer. A medical professional inserts an instrument into the vagina so she can see the cervix and then uses a brush or cotton-tipped swab to collect cells from the cervix. This specimen is sent to a cytology lab, where a cytotechnologist looks at the cells under a microscope. If any abnormalities are detected, the test is routed to a pathologist for further evaluation.

Who needs a Pap test?

- Recommendations for the timing and frequency of Pap testing continue to evolve. Major changes were published in 2012, and current recommendations can be found at the American College of Obstetricians and Gynecologists, the American Society for Colposcopy and Cervical Pathology, the US Preventive Services Task Force, and the American Cancer Society.

- Initial Pap testing is now recommended at age 21, regardless of when a woman becomes sexually active.
- Women 21–29 should have a Pap test every 3 years.
- Women 30–65 should be tested with either a Pap test alone every 3 years, or a Pap test and an HPV co-test every 5 years.
- Women with abnormal results, previous cervical cancer, impaired immune systems, or other complicating factors need to discuss their recommended Pap testing frequency with their healthcare providers.

How do I prepare for a Pap test?

- Do not have sex, douche, use tampons, or use any vaginal cream, gel, or foam (including spermicides) for two days prior to your Pap test.
- Schedule your Pap test for a time when you should not be having your period.

Can cervical cancer be cured?

- Yes. Many cervical cancers are caught early and can be cured with treatment.

Can you be reinfected?

- Cancer can recur.

What are the basic stages of cervical cancer?

- Stage 0: The cancer is found only in the top layer of cells in the tissue that lines the cervix. Stage 0 is also called carcinoma in situ.
- Stage I: The cancer has invaded the cervix beneath the top layer of cells. Abnormal cells are found only in the cervix.
- Stage II: The cancer extends beyond the cervix into nearby tissues. It extends to the upper part of the vagina. The cancer does not invade the lower third of the vagina or the pelvic wall (the lining of the part of the body between the hips).
- Stage III: The cancer extends to the lower part of the vagina. It also may have spread to the pelvic wall and nearby lymph nodes.
- Stage IV: The cancer has spread to the bladder, rectum, or other parts of the body.

What is the treatment?

- Multiple treatments exist, and type of treatment depends on staging of the disease. Thanks to Pap tests, many cervical cancers are discovered at stage 0 or stage I and therefore are easily treated. Treatments include:
- Surgery: In stage 0 (very early cancer), surgical treatment can be performed that leaves the uterus intact, allowing the possibility of future childbearing. More advanced stages may require removal of the uterus, fallopian tubes, and ovaries.
- Chemotherapy.
- Radiation.
- Combination of any of the above methods.

How about alternative therapies?

- No herbal or home remedies have been proven to eliminate cervical cancer.

Are there long-term consequences?

- Infertility, if there is scarring from the treatment; more common at stage I and beyond.
- Death: an estimated 4,000 women die from cervical cancer each year in the United States.

When are you contagious?

- Any time you are infected with HPV, regardless of symptoms, you are contagious. However, you can only transmit the virus, not cervical cancer itself.
- Latex male condoms can reduce but not eliminate transmission of HPV, since HPV is present on genital surfaces not covered with a condom.

How can I avoid getting cervical cancer?

- Abstinence or monogamy with a partner who has had no prior sexual partners will prevent getting HPV, which causes cervical cancer.
- HPV vaccines provide excellent prevention against cervical cancer as long as they are administered before the individual has become sexually active (in other words, the vaccine must be received before the individual has been exposed to HPV).
- HPV vaccines Gardasil and Cervarix prevent infection with HPV types 16 and 18, which cause 70% of cervical cancers.

- HPV vaccine Gardasil-9 prevents infection with HPV types 16, 18, 31, 33, 45, 52, and 58, which cause 90% of cervical cancers.

Frequently Asked Questions

➤ **How many abnormal Pap tests turn out to be invasive cancer?**
Out of 50 million Pap tests annually, roughly 2 million are abnormal, and only 11,000 are invasive cancers.

➤ **Does smoking cause cervical cancer?**
The human papilloma virus causes cervical cancer, but women with HPV who smoke have a higher incidence of cervical cancer than those with HPV who do not smoke.

➤ **Will my genital warts turn into cancer?**
Although the risk is not zero, it's very unlikely. Warts are caused by different strains of HPV than those that typically cause cancer.

➤ **If I have cervical cancer, does that count as an STI?**
Yes. We now know that cervical cancers are caused by HPV, although risk factors like smoking, weakened immune system, age over 40, and lack of regular Pap tests do contribute.

➤ **To catch HPV, do you have to have sex with multiple partners?**
No. Although your risk of any STI increases with the number of partners you have had, HPV is so widespread that you can easily contract it even from your first partner (unless you both have had no prior genital contact).

➤ **If I get an HPV vaccine, can I still get cervical cancer?**
Yes. The original Gardasil and Cervarix vaccines protect against the types of HPV that cause 70% of cervical cancers, so there is still the possibility of contracting the types of HPV that cause the other 30% of cervical cancers.

Similarly, Gardasil-9 protects against the types of HPV that cause 90% of cervical cancers, leaving a chance of catching the types of HPV that cause the remaining 10% of cervical cancers.

➤ **If I get an HPV vaccine, do I need to use condoms?**
Yes, absolutely. HPV vaccines protect well against HPV but do not protect against any other STIs.

➤ **Is the HPV vaccine safe?**
Yes. Between 2006 and 2015, over 70 million doses of Gardasil were administered in the United States. Our national reporting systems are open to the public, and there have been approximately 25,000 cases of "adverse events" related to the HPV vaccines, the majority of which are minor medical issues such as local redness, pain, or swelling at the site of vaccination, nausea, dizziness, or fainting. Eight percent of the reports of adverse events were considered serious (including blood clots, cancers, and death), but there is no pattern to suggest that these events were indeed caused by the vaccine.
Although relatively infrequent, there is an increased incidence of fainting within the first fifteen minutes after receiving a dose of Gardasil, so patients are advised to remain seated or lying down for that time frame.

➤ **Are there support groups for women who have cervical cancer?**
Absolutely! Cervical cancer awareness and support is increasing across the United States. Local, national, and online support groups offer helpful information and community, whether they are part of larger organizations, such as the American Cancer Society and the National Cervical Cancer Coalition, or foundations started by cervical cancer survivors, such as Tamika and Friends and its associated group, Cervivors.

Additional Information

American College of Obstetricians and Gynecologists
PO Box 70620
Washington, DC 20024-9998
1-800-673-8444
www.acog.org/publications/patient_education/bp163.cfm

American Sexual Health Association
PO Box 13827
Research Triangle Park, NC 27709
919-361-8400
www.ashasexualhealth.org/

Centers for Disease Control and Prevention
1600 Clifton Road
Atlanta, GA 30329-4027
1-800-CDC-INFO (1-800-232-4636), 1-888-232-6348 (TTY)
www.cdc.gov/cancer/cervical/

HPV Vaccine—Questions and Answers
www.cdc.gov/vaccines/vpd-vac/hpv/vac-faqs.htm

MedlinePlus
US National Library of Medicine
8600 Rockville Pike
Bethesda, MD 20894
1-888-FIND-NLM (1-888-346-3656) or 301-594-5983
www.nlm.nih.gov/medlineplus/cervicalcancer.html

National Cancer Institute
9609 Medical Center Drive
Bethesda, MD 20892-9760
1-800-4-CANCER (1-800-422-6237)
www.cancer.gov/cancertopics/types/cervical

National Cervical Cancer Coalition
www.nccc-online.org

Tamika and Friends, Inc.
www.tamikaandfriends.org

CHLAMYDIA

6: Tyler

Tyler winced as he finished urinating. "Ow! What the . . . ? Why is it hurting to pee? I guess I must have had too much to drink." Over the weekend, he had downed at least a twelve-pack of beer during an all-day fraternity party, not to mention the vodka that he and his friends had snuck into the game. Basketball season was always awesome, although the hangovers after the games weren't so much fun. Last weekend had been especially crazy, with the road trip to meet his college's cross-state rivals. To top it all off, Tyler had hooked up with his ex-girlfriend, Sierra, when she showed up at the party.

There had been one pretty embarrassing moment, however, when they had sex after the game. Tyler couldn't believe that he had drunk so much that it was difficult to keep an erection. He'd heard guys joke about "whiskey dick" but didn't imagine that it happened to nineteen-year-olds. Thank goodness Sierra was cool with him taking off the condom so he could feel more. After that, he had no problems.

He and Sierra had been together over the summer but had broken up during the second week of school. Tyler heard that she had dated some grad student who lived in her apartment complex, followed by a self-described computer geek. When he saw her at the party, Sierra said she missed Tyler and wanted to get back together. Tyler was far from wanting to get emotionally serious with anyone, but the idea of a steady girlfriend and predictable hookups was enticing. Tyler had had a few girlfriends in high school and during his freshman year of college, but this was his first girlfriend who didn't have any hangups about sex. Sierra was, as she said, "very comfortable with her body" and had taught Tyler quite a bit about sexual intimacy.

By the end of the day on Monday, Tyler had downed several bottles of water and a couple of sports drinks. He had to pee about once an hour from all those drinks, and it seemed to burn worse each time he went. As he fought the snow and ice while trekking across campus, he realized he was passing the Quack Shack—the university's health center. "I'd better get checked out," he thought. "But what am I going to tell them my problem is?" How embarrassing to say that he had a problem with peeing. Tyler had three older sisters who always joked about their tiny bladders and how often they had to stop on road trips to use the restroom. One time, all the siblings had given grief to the oldest sister, Bailey, about stopping every five minutes, only to find out later, when she became ill with a fever and chills, that she actually had a kidney infection. What if that happened to him? He had a term paper due in one class and a test in another this week. It was certainly not the time to get sick. So, Tyler decided to go into the health center and headed over to the scheduling area.

"Hi. Can I get an appointment today?," he asked.

"We don't have space left for routine visits today. What kind of problem are you having?," asked the cute young woman behind the counter.

"I, uh, think I've got a kidney problem."

"Do you have any fever, chills, nausea, or vomiting?," she asked as she typed into her computer.

"No."

"Back pain?"

"No."

"Burning when you urinate?"

"Yes." There it was, without him having to say it. Phew.

"Discharge?"

Tyler flushed to the roots of his hair. "No!"

"Okay, then. Our urgent care spots are full for today, but it looks like we can get you in tomorrow morning at ten fifteen. Please fill out your forms online before you arrive. Here is your reminder card with the website." She handed him a small card. "If you get worse during the night, you can call our nurse triage line and they can help. Otherwise, just drink plenty of fluids, and we'll see you back here tomorrow."

"Thanks," said Tyler. And then he thought, "Well, it can't be that big of a deal, since they're having me come back in the morning. Maybe I'll wake up tomorrow and be back to normal anyway."

Tyler's mind went back to all his tasks for the week ahead. He was totally behind on his paper for English, so he'd better head to the library before he went home. He flushed again when he remembered the young woman at the desk asking if he had any "discharge." How embarrassing. It's not like he had an STI or something. His crazy roommate had actually gotten gonorrhea last year after a particularly wild frat party, but that had been totally different. Now *there* was someone complaining of a "discharge." Joe had whined about catching the clap from this "loose girl" he had slept with. That poor overweight young woman was desperate for attention. Tyler guessed that she had hooked up with half the guys in his frat. He didn't even know her name, but they all called her "Afternoon Delight." Tyler thought that catching something had served Joe right for not being pickier about his sex partners.

A girl like Sierra, on the other hand, would never give you a disease. She kept herself very together. Sierra always looked like she had just stepped out of some fancy magazine, with her clothes always perfectly in style with the current fashions. As he thought about Sierra being back in his life, he fished around for his cell phone to text her.

"Hey, are you done with classes?"

"Yes! I finished an hour ago and I'm starving! Want to order pizza and study at my place?," Sierra texted back almost immediately.

"Sure. On my way," Tyler replied. He laughed to himself as he realized how quickly he had slipped back into the whole boyfriend role.

After dinner, they went back to her apartment and actually did a couple of hours of studying. Unfortunately, Tyler needed to get up and go to the bathroom constantly, and the burning was not getting better. Tyler decided to head back to his room.

"What, you're not staying the night?," Sierra pouted. Suddenly, Tyler remembered how possessive Sierra had always been with his time. It was enough to irritate him into an abrupt response.

"No, I'm not. I just want to get a good night's sleep in my own bed," he snapped. Sierra looked crushed, and he regretted sounding so harsh. He quickly added, "Honestly, I think I might have a kidney infection or something. It kind of hurts to pee. Have you ever had something like that?"

"A kidney infection? Do you mean a bladder infection?," she asked.

"What's the difference?"

"I don't know exactly, but once last year I had to pee all the time, and it kind of hurt when I went. The doctor said it was a bladder infection, and after I took antibiotics for a couple of days I was fine. Are you going to the doctor?," she asked.

Tyler felt kind of relieved to tell her about it. "Yeah, I've got an appointment for the morning. Would you believe that they, uh, they asked me if I had a 'discharge'—you know, like I had an STI or something. Isn't that ridiculous?" Tyler managed a laugh as he glanced sideways to catch Sierra's response. It appeared that this was not what she wanted to hear.

"What is that supposed to mean?," she demanded. "Who were you with while we were broken up?" Sierra glared at him across the room.

Tyler recoiled. "Whoa… slow down. You were the one dating a bunch of people, but I'm not accusing you of anything. I think I just drank too much beer over the weekend and got a bladder infection or whatever."

Sierra chewed on her lip for a minute, then came over and sat down next to Tyler. "I'm sorry. I'm sure you're right. When is your appointment?"

"Tomorrow morning at ten fifteen, right after my English class," Tyler replied.

"Oh, good. You at least got a morning appointment. Do you want to meet me for lunch afterward? We could grab some sandwiches or something."

"Sounds great." Tyler gave her a quick kiss and promised to text her after the appointment.

The next morning, Tyler was relieved that it didn't seem to hurt so much when he went to the bathroom. He almost blew off his appointment but decided he might as well go in, since he wasn't completely back to normal. Tyler had forgotten to fill out the online forms before he arrived, but managed to finish them on his phone while he waited to be called to the exam room. Finally, they called his name. The medical assistant took his weight, temperature, pulse, and blood pressure, entering the information into her tablet. She scrolled down, and then she looked up and began to ask him questions.

"So, what brings you in to see the doctor today?," she asked brightly.

"Can she not read what I entered?," he wondered. Tyler considered a sarcastic reply, but instead muttered, "I think I have a bladder infection."

"When did your symptoms start?"

"Yesterday morning."

"Do you have burning when you urinate?"

"Yes."

"Any urgency or increased frequency of urinating?"

"Kind of, I guess," he said.

She continued, "Any fever, nausea, or vomiting?"

"No."

"Any discharge from your penis?," she asked without even looking up from her tablet.

"No!," he exclaimed, feeling the flush return to his face. What was it with these people and "discharge"?

"Any unprotected intercourse in the recent past?," she inquired.

"No."

"Okay, then. Head down the hall to the last door on the left. In the bathroom, there are urine sample cups. Follow the instructions on the wall poster to give us a clean-catch specimen, please. Then come back to this room, change into this gown, and the doctor will be in after she looks at your urine under the microscope. Per our office's medical-legal policy, a medical assistant will also come in the room to assist her and to serve as a chaperone if Dr. Lampert needs to examine your groin area. Any questions?" She rattled off this routine, as she clearly must have done a hundred times per week.

Tyler initially felt more relaxed as he headed down the hallway toward the bathroom, glad he would get some answers. More relaxed that is, until it hit him that the medical assistant had just referred to his doctor as a *she*. Oh man, a female doctor. Wait—*and a chaperone?* Would that be another woman? Surely the doctor wouldn't have to examine him, would she? What was that part about changing into a gown? He felt his heart racing.

Quickly he followed the instructions on the wall, cleaning his penis with the special wipe and then catching his urine in the cup midstream. Of course, it didn't seem to hurt too much now as he peed. "Great, I'm here for nothing." Just like taking your car into the mechanic for a funny noise, and it disappears when you arrive at the garage. "Oh well, if my urine checks out okay, then we shouldn't have to do anything else, I suppose." Tyler placed the sample in the basket as the sign instructed and headed back to the exam room.

He looked at the gown. Should it be open at the front or the back? He decided to leave his boxers on and wear the gown open at the front like a jacket. He got changed and sat on the table to wait. Unfortunately, it took twenty minutes until the doctor walked in. Plenty of time for Tyler to think back over last weekend.

The door popped open, and a woman wearing scrubs stepped in, along with a young man in scrubs who looked no older than Tyler.

"Hi, I'm Dr. Lampert," she said, "and this is Matt, another of our medical assistants." Tyler was relieved that Matt seemed a bit disengaged from the whole process, and was standing off to the side looking at his notebook. The young doctor seemed friendly enough, and Tyler noticed she was wearing a splint.

"What happened to your arm?," he asked, shifting the focus onto her.

"I fell off my mountain bike last week and sprained my wrist. Thank goodness it was my left arm, or I could never function," replied Dr. Lampert.

"Cool," Tyler replied, then quickly added, "I mean cool that you were mountain biking, not that you got hurt."

The doctor grinned. "No problem, I knew what you meant. Do you bike too?"

"I love single-track," he affirmed. "My favorite place to ride is the greenbelt behind Mountain Vista."

"No kidding? That's where I fell, past the old bridge, where the switchbacks start."

"And all the big rocks," Tyler added.

"Yes, the big slippery rocks," laughed the doctor. "I guess that explains my problem, so let's move on to yours. Your record says you've had some burning when you pee for the last few days."

Tyler felt his pulse racing again. But at least she was looking at his records, he thought. "Yes. It started yesterday morning, but it seems a little better today," he replied.

"No fever that you were aware of?"

"No."

"And no nausea or back pain?," she asked, taking note of his responses.

"None. Just the burning."

"Got it. Have you had sex with any new partners?"

"Well, I did just get back together with my girlfriend. But no one new." Tyler smiled.

Dr. Lampert looked at him intently: "Have you used condoms every time?"

Now Tyler was not smiling. "Well, I guess not a hundred percent."

"And you haven't noted any discharge?," she pressed.

"No, despite being asked that a million times here," Tyler retorted.

"Sorry, but you'd be amazed how answers sometimes change when they're asked more than once," she said, raising an eyebrow.

She put his chart down, stood up, and reached for gloves, which went on easily despite her splint. "I've already looked at your urine sample, and this doesn't look like a typical urinary tract infection."

"Meaning what?," Tyler interrupted.

"Meaning you had some white blood cells, which indicate inflammation, but no bacteria. Therefore, the most common cause of your painful urination would be urethritis, an inflammation of the tube that carries the urine from your bladder out your penis. We need to check you for any sexually transmitted infections, to see if that's what's causing your symptoms. We will check your urine sample for chlamydia and gonorrhea, but those test results won't be back until tomorrow. Let me take a quick look at you now, to make sure we are not missing any lumps, bumps, or lesions from other STIs, okay?"

Dr. Lampert started by firmly thumping on his back with the side of her fist, asking, "Does this hurt? This is where your kidneys live." Then she told him, "Lie back on the exam table, please." Tyler leaned back but stayed propped up on his elbows. Dr. Lampert prodded his abdomen, and then quickly examined his genitals.

"All right, you survived," Dr. Lampert said with a smile, "and everything appears normal. Let us step out so you can get dressed. Then I'll be back in to give you a prescription and discuss our game plan."

Tyler hopped off the table and grabbed his clothes. He quickly dressed and sat down in the chair. Before he'd even had time to process what the doctor had said so far, there was a knock on the door and Dr. Lampert came back in.

"Okay, Tyler. I've got a prescription here for you for a drug called azithromycin. You'll take two five-hundred-milligram pills together at one time today, and that is a complete treatment. You should be feeling better in a couple of days. We'll have your test results back in two to three days. The urine culture takes three days, but I really think that will be negative. Guys just don't get urinary tract infections as often as girls do, because their urethra is farther away from their anus, so the bacteria can't move as easily to set up an infection. You most likely have a chlamydia infection, which is sexually transmitted. Therefore, if your test comes back positive for chlamydia, your girlfriend will need treatment too." Dr. Lampert paused a moment, sensing that Tyler would have a comment.

"Doctor," he began, "no offense, but I just really doubt this is an STI. Sierra is the only, uh, person that I've ever been with, and she's, well, a nice girl." Tyler knew that sounded lame, but really, a polished, chic sorority girl like Sierra having an STI?

Dr. Lampert took a big breath and let it out slowly. "Tyler, I have no doubt that Sierra is a great girl. But I'm going to tell you the rules of life that I see enacted every day, okay?"

Tyler shrugged. "Sure."

"Okay, here they are. My three rules to live by. One, everybody has a disease or an infection. Two, everybody lies. Three, young women are fertile. Now, let me clarify. Number one, everybody has disease or infection. Nearly ninety percent of adults have oral herpes, which can be transmitted through oral sex, and no one seems to consider this a risk. Many, many people have other diseases like chlamydia or the wart virus but have literally *no* symptoms, so they believe they have no disease, and therefore I guess technically they're not lying, but ultimately they are still passing along infection."

She continued, "Many people do know when they have genital herpes, because it hurts. Others truly have a silent infection. Regardless, it's quite embarrassing to tell someone you're in love with that you've got herpes, so many people just don't. Especially if they haven't had an outbreak in a while. They may be telling themselves that they aren't contagious anymore, but that unfortunately isn't true. As for number three, I've seen many undergrads in here in tears because they're pregnant, even though they were on the pill or using condoms. Condoms break, and it's too often at the exact moment the girl is ovulating. The pill is ninety-nine percent effective when it's taken at the same exact time every day, but lots of young women take it whenever they wake up or go to bed, which changes by many hours on the weekends versus the weekdays. At the end of the day, my rules stand." Tyler just looked at her somewhat disbelievingly.

Dr. Lampert went on, "So, the test we are performing on your urine is for chlamydia and gonorrhea; it'll be back in two days. If the chlamydia portion is positive, you'll already be receiving treatment for that, but if the gonorrhea part is positive, that will require a different antibiotic. If either one is positive, your girlfriend will need treatment. She will have to see her physician in order to be prescribed the appropriate treatment."

Tyler sat there a minute. He took the prescription that Dr. Lampert extended to him.

"Do you really think this is chlamydia, or whatever? Wouldn't she know if she had a problem? And what is chlamydia, anyway?," he asked.

Dr. Lampert shook her head as she replied, "Most people who have chlamydia are completely asymptomatic—no discharge, no pain, no clue. That's why this infection gets spread so easily. It's actually not hard to treat—simply a short round of antibiotics. It's really important to treat it, though, even when people aren't bothered by any symptoms, because down the road, untreated chlamydia infections can cause scarring of a woman's fallopian tubes and therefore cause infertility. It's thought that a majority of infertility is due to this very problem. As for your question about what exactly it is—chlamydia is kind of in between a virus and bacteria. It's bigger than a virus particle, but it lives inside of human cells. That's why it takes a certain type of antibiotic to kill it, one that enters the cells. Does that help?"

Tyler sighed. "I guess so. How do you know people have it if they don't know themselves, and they don't have symptoms?"

"Good question. The answer is that any time a woman comes in for her annual exam, which we require in order to get a prescription of birth control pills, we ask if she has had any new sexual partners. If the answer is yes, we routinely test for all STIs, including the test I just used on you. You'd be amazed how many come back positive. Speaking of that, I should offer you complete testing for sexually transmitted infections since you had unprotected sex—even though it was just with one person, one time. It's certainly better to be safe than sorry. We can draw your blood today and check for syphilis, HIV, hepatitis C, and herpes antibodies. If you'd like to do that, head downstairs to the lab when we are finished."

Tyler put his hand up in the universal sign for stop. "No, thanks. I appreciate what you've said, but I just don't think I need it. I will go ahead and get this antibiotic and take it, but I'll wait until my test comes back before I worry about any other STIs. If it's positive, then I'll come back and get my blood drawn, okay?"

Dr. Lampert shrugged her shoulders. "That's your choice, of course. I'll go ahead and order the lab request so it will be in your records. Think about it, and think about asking your girlfriend to get tested as well. I encourage you to use condoms if you're going to have sex, both for disease prevention and for extra contraception, even if she's on the pill."

Dr. Lampert finished documenting her notes in the electronic medical record. She stood and opened the exam room door. "Check out down the hall to the right, and they'll direct you to the pharmacy. Let me know if this doesn't take care of your symptoms."

Tyler checked out and got his prescription filled at the pharmacy. There was a soda machine in the waiting area, and he grabbed a drink so he could take his medicine. At least they're a reasonable size, he thought, as he popped the two pills and downed them with the soda. His cell phone chirped as he headed out of the building. Yep, right on cue, it was Sierra texting him to arrange a place for lunch.

They met at a sandwich shop by the student center. "Well, how did it go? Was it a bladder infection after all?," Sierra asked as they sat down with their lunches.

Tyler wasn't sure how to answer. "Well, the doctor wasn't sure, but she gave me some antibiotics and took some tests. To be honest, she made a big deal about both of us getting tested for STIs if we are going to . . . be together."

Tyler took a big bite of his sandwich, waiting to see what Sierra's response would be. He was afraid she would be offended or defensive. Instead, she was completely unconcerned. "Well, I get annual checkups for the pill, so I know I'm fine. Did you get everything checked?," she asked.

"Uh, no, not everything. Besides, you know you're the only one I've fully hooked up with, so if you're clear, so am I." Tyler thought back to Dr. Lampert's rules. Was Sierra lying, or could she have given him some infection unknowingly? More likely, he just had a bladder infection, and the medicine would clear it up. He cheered up, and they spent the rest of their lunch planning their upcoming weekend.

The next morning, Tyler awoke after a good night's sleep feeling great. It didn't hurt to go to the bathroom, and he generally seemed to have more energy. In fact, Tyler pretty much forgot about the infection until Friday morning, when he got a text from the health center alerting him that he had a secure message. He quickly logged on to his university health services account, entered his student ID, and clicked on his message.

> Tyler,
>
> Hope you are feeling better. Your test came back positive for chlamydia, as I had suspected. Fortunately, your urine was negative for gonorrhea, so the antibiotic I prescribed should have cured your infection, but your girlfriend will need to come in to get treated so you don't keep passing this back and forth. Please come in and get bloodwork done to check for all the other STIs, as we discussed. You can go straight to the lab, and we will send you another secure message with the results in a couple of days. Attached is a handout that should answer most of your questions about this infection, but let us know if you have any questions.
>
> Best wishes,
> Dr. Lampert

Tyler was speechless. "I have chlamydia? Could the test be wrong?" He opened the attachment and scanned through the information, most of which appeared to be what Dr. Lampert had already shared with him, but he wasn't really focusing.

Tyler put away his cell phone. He shook his head, trying to process the information but still unable to believe it. "Man, oh man, my first STI. And I hope my very last." Suddenly, everything the doctor said was spinning around in his head. What if he did have another infection that he didn't know about? What if it was HIV, or hepatitis, or that wart virus? Gross! He changed directions and headed back toward the health center. Why hadn't he just gotten his blood drawn while he was there? What was he thinking that day? He certainly wanted his blood drawn now.

He had said that Sierra was such a "nice girl." Well, here's one nice girl who had been "nice" to one guy too many. Since he had never had sex with anyone besides Sierra, Tyler was now completely sure that Sierra was the one who had given him this infection. So much for the bonus that she didn't have any hangups about sex. That had seemed so cool, but now Tyler realized it was not exactly a perk.

The doctor's words echoed in his brain. "Everyone has a disease or an infection. Everyone lies. Young women are fertile." He remembered Sierra's reassurance that she'd been tested and was "fine." Apparently that was before she'd had sex with someone carrying chlamydia and who knows what else. "Time for some new testing, Sierra," he thought. He started to text her, wondering as he typed if he could control his building anger. Tyler deleted his unfinished, unsent message.

Although he was extremely upset, deep down Tyler knew that some of his anger was misplaced. He was also really mad at himself. After all, he was the one who asked to remove the condom. How stupid was that? And Sierra had been very upfront that she was not a virgin. If Sierra had no symptoms, was it really her fault that she gave him an STI? While his bruised ego still pointed the finger at Sierra, the logical part of Tyler's brain was telling him to cool off before he made a rash decision about their relationship.

"First things first," Tyler decided. "I'll get my blood drawn at the health center, and make sure we're only dealing with one silent infection. I don't even have all the facts yet." Tyler stuffed his phone in his backpack, pulled his hat down to shield his ears from the wind, and hurried off.

7: Sofia

SOFIA PROUDLY SCANNED THE boutique, her eyes soaking in all the exquisite clothing. "I'm so glad you finally had a chance to stop by and check out my store. Look at these gorgeous Italian leather jackets," she gushed to her best friend and roommate, Erica. "With my employee discount, I can actually afford one."

"Lucky you," said Erica enviously. "My job at the club certainly wouldn't earn enough to cover it."

"Maybe not, but at least your job keeps you looking great no matter what you wear," Sofia shot back. Both girls laughed. Roommates since their freshman year in college, Sofia and Erica loved to tease each other about their chosen professions. Sofia planned to be a fashion designer, and Erica hoped to own her own fitness center. As recent graduates, they were thankful that both had landed jobs in their fields. Erica worked as a personal trainer at the busiest fitness center in town. Sofia was the assistant manager at Trixie's Boutique.

"Maybe one of your rich clients will sign up for a bunch of sessions, and you can splurge on something here. Really, though, not everything is super expensive. Look, how about one of these cute purses?," Sofia said, holding up a brightly colored bag. "Aren't these great?"

Erica slipped the purse straps over her shoulder, striking a pose to model the bag for Sofia. "How does this work with my outfit?," she joked.

Sofia chastised, "Now come on, nothing in here is going to match your sweaty workout clothes and running shoes."

Erica had to agree. "These extra inside pockets for my cell phone and keys would be nice, and there is enough room that I could stuff in a sweatshirt."

"Please! Simply getting you to use any purse instead of a backpack would be an improvement," said Sofia. "Well, feel free to look around. Let me know if you see something that you like. I need to get back to the computer and finish a restocking order before I leave for my gynecologist appointment during my lunch break."

"Oh yeah, I forgot you had that today," said Erica. "Glad I came by early, so I didn't miss you."

"I certainly couldn't forget," replied Sofia. "I'm actually kind of nervous. I haven't been to the doctor since I got off the pill a few years ago. I'm dreading having a pelvic exam from someone new. You never know how that will be."

"Don't stress, it'll be okay. Didn't you tell me you're seeing Dr. Taylor? I've heard she's great," reassured Erica. "Besides, you don't have anything wrong, do you?"

"Actually, this will be my first time going to the doctor without having some kind of problem," said Sofia.

"So I guess this will make you a real grownup," teased Erica. "Next, you'll be headed to the accountant to pay taxes."

Sofia smiled. "Here's hoping I make enough money to do that."

A short time later, Sofia found herself seated on the end of an exam table, nervous but pleasantly distracted as she examined the unique style of her patient gown.

"Just toss it on over your head, leaving the sides open like a poncho," the nurse had instructed.

Sofia's fashion sense admired the gown's physical warmth, functionality, and even whimsy. "Someone found the perfect print for a gynecologist's office," thought Sofia, admiring the bright red ladies' hats, purses, and shoes that adorned the material. From the pastel colors of the waiting room to the beautiful quilt hanging on the wall in the exam room, this practice had obviously put effort into aesthetics that would appeal to women. "How nice to have insurance and be able to come here," Sofia mused, starting to relax.

The door opened, and a tall woman wearing black slacks and a wine-colored silk blouse with a stethoscope hanging around her neck strode purposefully into the room. "Hi, I'm Dr. Taylor." She offered a firm handshake and added, "And this is my medical assistant, Rhonda," nodding at the younger and equally tall woman in pink scrubs who had entered behind her.

"Hi, I'm Sofia. It's nice to meet you. My compliments to your interior designer," she added.

"Thanks for noticing," said Dr. Taylor with a brisk smile. "My partners and I want women to feel as comfortable as possible here, so we tried to make the office seem more feminine than sterile." The doctor quickly typed into the computer, still standing, and continued, "I see you're here for a well-woman exam, is that right?"

"Yes," answered Sofia. "I also was thinking about going back on the pill."

"Meaning you've taken a birth control pill before?," asked the doctor.

"Yes, I took one for a couple of years in high school and college," replied Sofia.

"Do you remember which one?"

"I don't recall the name of it. It was in a compact-style container, like makeup, if that helps," said Sofia.

"Did you have any problems with it?"

"No. I loved it, especially knowing exactly when my period was coming. Also, my periods were a whole lot lighter and I had less cramping," said Sofia.

"Then why did you stop taking it?," asked Dr. Taylor.

"Well, I broke up with my long-term boyfriend during my sophomore year of college, and when my prescription ran out, I never went back for an exam to refill it," answered Sofia.

"And what have you done for protection since then?"

Sofia shrugged. "I've only had sex a couple of times over the last few years, and I haven't been serious enough with anyone to think I needed to be back on the pill."

"What has changed now?," asked Dr. Taylor.

"I finally have a job where the benefits include insurance," smiled Sofia.

"That's understandable. Would you like to be tested for sexually transmitted infections?," the doctor asked. "I try to encourage anyone who has had a new sexual partner since their last exam to be checked for all STIs."

"Why not? If my insurance will cover it, go right ahead," answered Sofia.

Dr. Taylor nodded at her assistant, spritzed her hands with sanitizer, and began Sofia's exam. The doctor felt Sofia's neck, listened to her heart and lungs, and then asked her to lie back. "Your medical questionnaire says you have never had any concerns about a sexually transmitted infection," noted the doctor.

"I'd hope not," said Sofia. "Alex and I were both virgins when we started sleeping together."

"Alex was the long-term boyfriend you referred to earlier?," asked Dr. Taylor.

Sofia nodded her agreement. Dr. Taylor was examining her breasts now. "Although the major medical organizations currently disagree about the role of breast self-exams in cancer prevention, I still encourage my patients to periodically check their breasts during their morning shower," she said. "Start way up here in your armpit and cover the whole surface of each breast in circles. I know it may seem like it all feels lumpy, but you're looking for something that feels hard, or stuck, or just doesn't move with the rest of the breast tissue. Also, look at the skin. If you ever see any redness, dimpling, puckering, or a bruise that you can't explain, you need to come in and let me take a look at it, all right?"

Again, Sofia nodded. The doctor moved down to her abdomen and then walked around to the end of the table, sitting down to perform the pelvic exam. Rhonda handed gloves and then a speculum to the doctor. "This may be a bit uncomfortable," said Dr. Taylor, as she positioned the instrument. "Since you are over twenty-one, current recommendations are that we do a Pap test every three years during your twenties." The doctor took a swab from her assistant and deftly performed the exam as she spoke. "We will test your urine sample for chlamydia and gonorrhea, the most common bacterial sexually transmitted infections. Additionally, we will run blood tests for syphilis, hepatitis C, and HIV."

Dr. Taylor finished her exam and stood up to leave. "Rhonda will give you a minute to get dressed. Then she will come back in and draw your blood, plus I'll have her bring you some samples of your new pill and explain when to start. Did you have any other concerns?"

Sofia hesitated, but responded, "I assume that this isn't something you'd deal with, but since you asked, can you tell me what kind of doctor I should see for a painful heel? My right foot has been killing me every time I stand up."

Dr. Taylor glanced over at the chair where Sofia had neatly folded her clothes and placed her shoes. Nodding in that direction, Dr. Taylor responded, "If you're wearing high heels like that every day, it won't matter who you see for foot pain. Try wearing flats or wedges, preferably ones that have a rounded toe instead of those pointy ends." She looked at her assistant, adding, "Rhonda, please give Sofia contact information for the orthopedic group that we recommend."

"Flats with rounded toes? Oh brother," thought Sofia. "That would not be the style statement that Trixie's wants to project. I might as well wear Erica's running shoes. Oh well, maybe I'll check out the foot doctor anyway." Sofia had barely had time to get dressed when a knock on the door announced the return of the assistant.

"Are you ready?," asked Rhonda. "I just need to draw your blood for a few tests, and then I'll explain these," she said, placing a package of contraceptive pills on the counter. She skillfully wrapped Sofia's arm with a rubber tourniquet and soon had two tubes of blood collected. "We'll send you the results via email if everything is normal. If anything comes back abnormal, I'll give you a call."

Rhonda instructed, "Now, here is your birth control. You'll want to start these the Sunday after your next period begins. If your period starts on a Sunday, go ahead and start taking the pills that day. Otherwise, whatever day you have your period, wait until the Sunday of that week to begin the pill pack. We'll need to see you back here during your third cycle on the pill to make sure that everything is working for you and that you don't have any intolerable side effects."

"What kind of side effects would that be?," asked Sofia. "I don't remember having any problems with the pill when I took it in the past."

"Then, you should be fine," said Rhonda. "Some women complain about nausea, breast tenderness, or slight bleeding between periods. Usually those things disappear by the third cycle if people hang in there and keep taking the pills at the same time every day. Try hard not to miss any pills, because that not only makes it less effective for birth control, but it makes the side effects worse."

"What about weight gain?," asked Sofia.

"This particular pill isn't bad about fluid retention," said the nurse. "Truly, though, most contraceptive pills do not cause significant weight gain. In controlled studies, roughly a third of the people taking oral contraceptives will gain two to three pounds, and the rest stay the same or even lose weight. Here is our handout on the pill. If you have any more questions that this sheet doesn't cover, feel free to call and ask me. Our number is on the bottom."

"You all seem to have this down to a science," said Sofia, glancing at her watch. "Thanks for getting me in and out so quickly."

"I can't promise it every time, but we certainly try," smiled Rhonda. "We'll see you in three months."

A few days later, Sofia and Erica were sprawled on the couch in their apartment, with a half-eaten pizza in its cardboard box on the coffee table in front of them. Sofia raised her wine glass. "Here's to reliving our college days," she toasted. "When is the last time you and I were actually here by ourselves at the same time? I don't think we've shared a meal in weeks."

"If this is how we eat when we're together, we shouldn't do it very often, or I'd weigh a zillion pounds," said Erica. "What would my clients say if they saw me eating pizza and drinking beer?," she asked, returning the salute with her bottle of Corona.

"Oh, lighten up, Erica. They'd just say you're human. You know we don't eat junk very often anymore. So, catch me up on your life. Do you have any sexy new clients? Remember, you're in charge of my social life now. The last couple of guys I picked were pretty lame," said Sofia.

"Especially Mr. 'What's for Breakfast?'—don't you think?," taunted Erica.

Sofia groaned. "Come on, don't remind me. That whole night only happened because I'd had such a long dry spell with guys. Surely everyone's entitled to one drunken one-night stand. Oh man, I was sick for two days after that. Truly, I can't even remember his name. What was it, Joey?"

"Jake, not Joey. I wasn't the one doing tequila shots, so I remember quite clearly," said Erica.

"Okay, Jake, whatever. His name is now banished from this apartment, okay? Anyway, we established years ago that you have better taste in guys. Where is your man tonight?"

"Austin is working the late shift tonight. He offered to cover for someone who's sick," answered Erica. "Austin really is a sweetheart. I wish he had a brother for you, because his friends are either taken or definitely not your type. But let me think." Erica took another sip from her beer. "I did start training a cute lawyer this week. He's actually pretty fit already, and he wants to start doing triathlons."

"And he's single?," asked Sofia.

"Absolutely. He was telling me a sob story about how women don't want to date lawyers, just doctors—oh, hey, that reminds me. How did your doctor's appointment go the other day?," Erica inquired.

"Oh my gosh, I'm glad you asked," said Sofia, reaching for her phone. "I completely forgot that they left me a voice message this afternoon to call their office. I could have sworn the nurse said they would email the results, but I don't see anything here. Oh well, I'll call tomorrow and see what's up. Anyway, the appointment actually went quite smoothly. The office was decorated tastefully, which you know I loved. Everyone was very nice, and I was in and out in less than an hour."

"What a relief. Maybe I should try that office too."

The topic quickly drifted back to eligible guys, and Erica and Sofia debated the relative merits of potential dates until nearly midnight.

The next morning, Sofia used her hands-free phone to call Dr. Taylor's office as she drove to work.

"Women's Health Associates, this is Rhonda, how may I help you?," chirped the assistant.

"Hi, Rhonda, this is Sofia Davis. I was in for a physical the other day, and yesterday I received a voicemail to call the office. What's up?"

"Just a second, Sofia, let me pull up your records on the computer," said Rhonda.

Sofia sipped on her latte as she waited, looking around at the traffic.

"Okay, I've got it. Are you still there?," asked Rhonda.

"I'm here," replied Sofia.

"Dr. Taylor would like you to stop by this week to see me. Your STI test from your urine sample came back positive for both gonorrhea and chlamydia, so I'll need to give you a shot of one antibiotic and a prescription for a different one to clear them up. The good news is that your HIV, hepatitis, and syphilis tests all came back negative. Can you come in this morning?"

Sofia looked down at her skirt, where she'd just spilled some of her coffee while listening to Rhonda's report. "Sure," she said slowly. "What time did you want me to come in?"

"Actually, I had a last-minute cancellation for ten o'clock, if you can make it here that quickly."

"I'm just a few blocks away, so I'll come right over," said Sofia. She clicked off the call and grabbed for a napkin to blot her skirt. Rhonda had been so businesslike, so very matter-of-fact, that Sofia hadn't even questioned what she was saying. "This has to be wrong," thought Sofia. "I don't have any symptoms." Her mind went back and forth, thinking about the couple of guys she'd been with since she broke up with Alex three years ago. "No, this has to be a mistake," Sofia concluded as she parked and headed back into the beautiful office, this time completely oblivious to her surroundings.

Sofia checked in and was relieved the receptionist was expecting her. Before long, Rhonda, today wearing purple scrubs, came to the doorway and called her name. "Thanks for coming right over," said Rhonda. Sofia stepped through the door that Rhonda held open for her and followed her down the hall and into an exam room.

Rhonda opened a cabinet door and began drawing up a shot as Sofia sat down. "So, um, did I understand you to say that I have not one but two infections?," Sofia asked in disbelief. "I mean, there must be a mistake, because I don't have any symptoms at all."

Rhonda gave Sofia a sympathetic smile. "Most of the time, that's what we see. Some days it seems like we get as many positive results from our routine screenings as we do from people coming in with complaints of discharge."

"But two different infections? How is that possible?," asked Sofia.

"I'll give you information sheets on both infections that will explain more, but these two STIs show up together so often that it's recommended to either test or simply automatically treat for the other infection when one is positive. Think of it as bonus points," Rhonda tried to joke. "Seriously, though, consider yourself lucky. With antibiotics, both chlamydia and gonorrhea are completely cured. You certainly can't say that for herpes or warts, and we see those all the time too." Rhonda stepped across the room, helped Sofia to stand up, and prepared her hip for a shot.

"Oh gosh, in my hip? I haven't had a shot there since I was little," Sofia whimpered.

"Sorry. The hip muscle is bigger, so it works better for this shot, with less soreness or swelling than if we give it in the arm. Ready? This will sting for about a minute," she announced, swiftly delivering the injection.

"I'm sorry, but it's hard to believe that I have this—these—infections. I haven't had sex with anyone in over a month, and the time before that was practically a year ago," protested Sofia, reaching down to rub her burning hip.

"Did you use condoms?," asked Rhonda.

"Not the one last month. I'm embarrassed to admit it, but I was so drunk that I didn't care. I suppose I'm lucky I didn't get pregnant, on top of everything else. That night was a disaster any way you look at it," said Sofia, shaking her head in disgust.

"I'm sure you'll remember to always use condoms in the future," Rhonda said kindly.

"That's for sure," agreed Sofia.

"Well, at least you found out about the STIs. Since these infections often have no symptoms, a lot of people don't realize they have them until they develop a serious problem like infertility or pelvic inflammatory disease," said Rhonda.

Sofia's eyes widened. "Can this make me sterile?"

"Given your time frame, I doubt it. The shot I just gave you was ceftriaxone, and it should completely get rid of your gonorrhea. Here is a prescription for an oral antibiotic, azithromycin. The pharmacist will make you a liquid that you drink all at once, and then your chlamydia will be cured as well. You ought to contact any partners that you've had, so they can get tested and treated too. I'm sorry to rush, but why don't you read through these handouts, and then call me if I can answer any more questions for you, okay?"

"Just one last thing, if you don't mind. What are the chances that the test was wrong?," asked Sofia.

Rhonda smiled. "This is probably the one statistic that I know, because I get asked that all the time. The test is a DNA probe, with a sensitivity of up to ninety-eight percent and specificity between ninety-eight and ninety-nine percent for each infection. 'Sensitivity' means how often a test detects an infection when it is present, so this test finds the STI when it is there all but two percent of the time. 'Specificity' tells how often people without an infection get a negative result, so again this test is very accurate, not resulting in false positives more than one or two percent of the time. The chances of both of your tests appearing positive and actually being wrong is next to nothing. Does that help?"

Sofia shrugged. "It certainly sounds convincing."

"Okay then, you can head back down the hall and check out. I hope to be emailing you the results of your Pap test," Rhonda said, emphasizing the word "emailing."

"I can only hope I've scored enough 'bonus points' already for this visit. No offense, but I'd rather not get another phone call from you," replied Sofia wryly, tucking her information sheets and prescription into her purse and heading out the door.

Sofia slid into her car, but before she started it, she pulled out her cell phone. The first call was to Trixie's. "I'm so sorry, but I just accidentally spilled my latte all over my skirt. I need to run home and change, but I'll be there by eleven," Sofia told Marlee, the sales associate who answered the phone.

Tears fell as she drove out of the parking lot and headed back to her apartment. The next call was to her best friend.

"Hey, Sofia, what's up? I've got a client waiting for me at the pool, so I can't really talk right now," said Erica. "Sofia, are you crying? What's wrong?"

Between sniffs and a few sobs, Sofia poured out her story. "Remember how I said Dr. Taylor's office left me voicemail yesterday? When I called this morning, they asked me to come back in because I caught not one but *two* nasty infections from my fabulous one-night stand last month. Or at least I can only assume it was him, since I never had any symptoms. I guess it could even be from last year."

"What a jerk! Do you think he knew? Are you going to call him and tell him? And hey, what did you catch? Herpes?," fired Erica in rapid succession.

"No, it's gonorrhea and chlamydia, and at least they're both curable. Who knows if he was even aware that he had anything? As for calling him, the answer is absolutely no way. I don't ever want to see or speak to him again, and frankly, I don't even know if I could track him down."

"Oh, Sofia, you've got to tell him. What if he sleeps with someone else?," Erica protested. "Besides which, Austin mentioned last week that he saw Jake hanging out at his gym. I didn't see any reason to say anything, but I'm telling you now because I know that Austin could ask around and locate him for you."

"Oh, sure, and have Austin plus everyone he asks figure out that I've got STIs? No thanks, Erica. Please promise me you won't tell Austin. I'll die if anyone finds this out," begged Sofia.

"Look, I've really got to run over to the pool, my client is waiting for me," said Erica, evading a direct response. "I promise not to say anything for now. Let's talk more about it tonight after work, all right?"

"Erica, come on. I trusted you with this information, and I'm asking you not to tell anyone. I'll see you tonight."

"All right," agreed Erica, childishly crossing her fingers behind her back. "Hang in there, and we'll talk later."

Both young women hung up, sharing the same thought. "How can she not understand? We'll talk tonight, and she'll see the whole picture. I know she'll agree with me."

facts

Chlamydia Fact Sheet

What is it?

- Chlamydia is an atypical bacteria called Chlamydia trachomatis.
- Chlamydia can cause pinkeye, upper respiratory infections, rectal inflammation, and infections in the urinary tract and cervix.

How common is it?

- The CDC notes that the reported cases in the United States exceeded 1 million for the first time in 2006, and unfortunately that trend has continued, with reported infections exceeding 1.4 million in 2012.
- Because it is silent up to 70% of the time, chlamydia is largely unreported, and yet it is one of the most widespread sexually transmitted infections in the United States.

- The CDC estimates that there are at least 2.86 million new cases of chlamydia annually in the United States.

- In 2014 the overall prevalence of chlamydial infection among people aged 14–39 was 1.7%, and in sexually active young women aged 14–24, the prevalence was 4.7%.

- Although chlamydia infections are common in all races, significant racial disparity exists: non-Hispanic black sexually active females aged 14–24: 13.5% (1 in 7); Mexican American sexually active females aged 14–24: 4.5% (1 in 22); non-Hispanic white sexually active females aged 14–24: 1.8% (1 in 55).

How do you get it?

- Chlamydia is transmitted through oral, vaginal, or anal sexual contact with an infected partner.

- It lives in semen and vaginal and respiratory secretions.

- Chlamydia can be passed to a baby during vaginal childbirth.

Where on your body do you get it?

- Women usually have infections in the cervix or urinary tract.

- Men get infections in the urethra or epididymis.

- Eye, mouth, and anus infections can occur in either sex.

How do I know if I have it?

- 50% of men and up to 75% of women are asymptomatic, so they only know they have chlamydia if they choose to get tested.

- Tests are conducted from a urine sample or from fluid collected from the cervix or penis with a swab.

- There is no readily available blood test for chlamydia.
- Pregnant women are routinely screened for chlamydia.
- All sexually active women should be screened at their annual exam.
- Infertile couples may discover that past chlamydia infections caused scarring of the woman's fallopian tubes.
- Men can have painful swelling of the scrotum from epididymitis.

What does it look like?

- Normal anatomy, or mild red irritation of the cervix or penis, with or without a gray to white discharge.

What does it feel like?

- Usually, people are unaware they have chlamydia.
- If symptoms are present, they include discharge (penile or vaginal) and burning with urination.
- Advanced infection can cause pelvic inflammatory disease (PID), which causes intense pelvic and abdominal pain.

How long does it last?

- Asymptomatic chlamydia infections can silently last for months or years until treated with appropriate antibiotics (which can happen serendipitously with treatment for an upper respiratory infection).
- Active symptoms can appear within one to three weeks from exposure.

- Symptoms resolve quickly with antibiotic treatment.

Can it be cured?

- Yes. Antibiotics can completely eliminate the bacteria, although they will not remove any damage done by chlamydia (such as scarring of the fallopian tubes).

Can you be reinfected?

- Yes. Prior episodes of chlamydia infection offer no protection. Reinfection is very common, especially when a partner is not fully treated.

- Each subsequent infection with chlamydia significantly increases the risk of long-term consequences.

What is the treatment?

- Antibiotics recommended to treat chlamydia include azithromycin, doxycycline, erythromycin, and ofloxacin.

How about alternative therapies?

- None have been proven to eliminate chlamydia.

Are there long-term consequences?

- 20%–40% of untreated chlamydia infections will go on to cause pelvic inflammatory disease (PID).

- PID causes scarring and blockage of fallopian tubes, causing an estimated 100,000 women to become infertile each year in the United States.

- Approximately 12% of women are infertile after a single episode of PID, almost 25% after two episodes, and over 50% after three or more episodes.

- PID scarring can also cause ectopic or tubal pregnancy (pregnancy occurring outside the uterus), which is potentially life threatening.

- PID can lead to chronic pelvic pain.

- Newborns exposed to chlamydia through the birth canal can develop serious eye infections or pneumonia in the first few weeks to months of life.

- Women with chlamydia infection are up to 5 times more likely to become infected with the HIV virus if exposed.

When are you contagious?

- Any time you are infected with chlamydia, regardless of symptoms.

- Even while using a condom. Latex male condoms can reduce but not eliminate transmission of chlamydia.

How do I avoid getting chlamydia?

- Abstaining from oral, vaginal, and anal sex will prevent getting chlamydia.

- Consistently using latex male condoms will reduce but not eliminate the risk of getting chlamydia.

- Having sex only in an exclusively monogamous relationship in which both partners have tested negative (or both have been successfully treated) will prevent chlamydia.

If I have chlamydia, how do I avoid giving it to my partner?

- If you have already had sex with your partner, abstain from oral, vaginal, and anal sex until a week after both you and your partner have been treated with antibiotics.

- If your partner has been tested and is negative, and you have not already had sex with him or her, wait one week after you have completed your antibiotic treatment before having oral, vaginal, or anal intercourse.

Can chlamydia be transmitted between homosexual partners?

- Rectal, oral, and urethral chlamydia infections can occur in homosexual male partners.

- Transmission via sex toys theoretically may occur.

- The possibility of female-to-female genital transmission is unclear, as there is a high incidence of lesbians having past or ongoing heterosexual contact (which makes pure female-to-female transmission rates uncertain).

Frequently Asked Questions

➤ **Is chlamydia the same as gonorrhea? Aren't they both "the clap"?**
No. The symptoms are often identical, but chlamydia and gonorrhea are caused by different bacteria, so they require treatment with different antibiotics.

➤ **Will penicillin cure chlamydia?**
No. To kill chlamydia, the antibiotic must enter the cell, which penicillin cannot do.

➤ **Can you get chlamydia from a toilet seat?**
No.

➤ **Can you have chlamydia and gonorrhea at the same time?**
Yes, this happens commonly.

Additional Information

American College of Obstetricians and Gynecologists
PO Box 70620
Washington, DC 20024-9998
1-800-673-8444
www.acog.org/publications/patient_education/bp009.cfm

American Sexual Health Association
PO Box 13827
Research Triangle Park, NC 27709
919-361-8400
www.ashasexualhealth.org/

Centers for Disease Control and Prevention
1600 Clifton Road
Atlanta, GA 30329-4027
1-800-CDC-INFO (1-800-232-4636), 1-888-232-6348 (TTY)
www.cdc.gov/STD/chlamydia/default.htm

MedlinePlus
US National Library of Medicine
8600 Rockville Pike
Bethesda, MD 20894
1-888-FIND-NLM (1-888-346-3656) or 301-594-5983
www.nlm.nih.gov/medlineplus/chlamydiainfections.html

GONORRHEA

8: Kiara

Kiara tried in vain to find a comfortable sitting position on the exam table. The waistband on her leggings seemed to dig into her lower belly, while abdominal cramps sent spasms of stabbing pain through her torso. Fever and body aches made her break out in a cold sweat, soaking her tunic top. "This has to be appendicitis," Kiara moaned to her best friend, Madison.

"At least you look cute in your new outfit," teased Madison.

"Cute doesn't help if I feel like my insides are exploding," replied Kiara.

"Try and use your yoga breathing, Kiara," advised Madison. "Remember how we learned to cleanse our minds with deep breaths and channel our energy?"

"All my energy appears to be focusing on pain, and I'd say it's channeling quite effectively," she snapped.

"Okay, then, at least change into that robe they left you," suggested Madison tolerantly.

"Quite the fashion statement, isn't it?," mocked Kiara, as she pulled on the patient gown, which was a thin white robe covered in blue polka dots.

"Yeah, right. It would be much cooler if you got to wear scrubs," offered Madison.

Kiara grimaced. "Madi, I don't mean to be such a wimp, but this really, really hurts."

"Hang in there, Kiara, I'm pretty sure you're next," reassured Madison.

"That's what they've been saying for the last hour," whined Kiara.

"I know, but it sounds like someone is having a heart attack, best that I can figure." Madison leaned forward, continuing in a conspiratorial low voice, "I heard them talking about an abnormal EKG, and then they asked for the cardiology attending. It's almost like in our acting class last month, when we were performing scenes out of *Grey's Anatomy*. At least that taught us a bunch of the lingo that they use in real emergency rooms."

"Well, it doesn't need to be Dr. McDreamy for me. I'd take any doctor right this minute, as long as they give me something for this pain," responded Kiara through gritted teeth. "This feels like a prison or something. When will they come?" Her eyes searched the tiny exam room. As if on cue, the curtain slid open, and a tired-looking but very attractive young man with rumpled green scrubs and a five o'clock shadow pulled the curtain shut as he sank onto the stool next to the bed. "Hi, I'm Dr. Knight. I understand you're having some abdominal pain today."

"That's the understatement of the century," exclaimed Kiara. "I'm dying here. Can you please get me some pain medicine? I've been lying here writhing in pain for over an hour."

"I'm sorry, but we've gotten slammed with patients all day long. I need to examine you before I can get you anything for pain, so I'll try and get through your history as quickly as possible, okay?," the doctor said.

"Fire away," consented Kiara.

Looking at her chart, Dr. Knight rattled off, "You're twenty-two years old, with no major medical problems like diabetes, seizures, asthma, or any other chronic illness, right?"

"We think she's got appendicitis, Dr. Knight," interjected Madison.

Dr. Knight looked up, apparently noticing Kiara's friend for the first time. Madison was squeezed between the exam table and the curtain, looking totally out of place in the hectic emergency room with her chic dress and perfectly straightened black hair. "That's a possibility," he said. Looking back at Kiara, he continued, "Have you had any abdominal surgeries? Appendix, gallbladder, or any gynecological procedures?"

"No," they answered in unison.

"Do you take any medicines on a regular basis?," he continued, noting Kiara's responses on the chart.

"Just my allergy nose spray," Kiara managed to answer.

"And your birth control pill," Madison added helpfully.

"Any allergies to medications?," Dr. Knight continued, focusing on Kiara.

"Penicillin. Come on, it's right there on her admissions bracelet," answered Madison in frustration.

"I'm sorry, but I really need to ask all these questions. I'm trying to help your friend here. Please let her answer," he said, irritation in his voice. "Kiara, what was your reaction to penicillin?"

"My mom says I had a really bad rash everywhere, and they were worried I would stop breathing," she answered.

"Fair enough, that sounds like a true drug allergy," he noted, as Madison rolled her eyes.

"Okay, last set of questions. I see that your last period started ten days ago. Are your periods regular?"

"Usually. I've had some spotting lately," Kiara answered.

"Any chance you could be pregnant?," Dr. Knight asked.

"No. Remember, I'm on the pill," Kiara said between held breaths. "And besides, as you should see in my chart, I just finished my period last week."

"Any new sexual partners within the last couple of months?," he inquired.

"Yes, not that I see why that matters," said Kiara.

"Did you use condoms?," he inquired.

"No, *she's on the pill*," Madison emphasized, as Kiara shook her head no.

"Have you ever had an STI?," asked the doctor.

There was a pause. "I had chlamydia once a couple of years ago, but that's all," answered Kiara quietly, looking away from her friend.

"Chlamydia? When did you have that?," interjected Madison, looking at Kiara with surprise. "Who gave you that?"

"Any vaginal discharge?," Dr. Knight continued, ignoring the comment.

"Honestly, I don't know. I'm just in pain," Kiara complained, also disregarding her friend's questions.

"Okay, let's talk about your pain. Obviously, it's in your lower belly. Is it steady or coming in waves?"

"No, it's not going away. It's steady," she answered.

"Any nausea, vomiting, or diarrhea?"

"A little nausea, yes."

"When did it start?," Dr. Knight asked.

"I've noticed an ache off and on the last few days, but then sometime this afternoon, it really kicked into high gear."

"Let's take a look at you," Dr. Knight said, setting his pen and chart down and standing beside Kiara.

"Finally," muttered Madison.

"Madison," Kiara warned with a look.

Dr. Knight audibly sighed, "It's all right, I know your friend is just worried about you. Do you want her to stay while I examine you?"

Kiara nodded her assent.

Dr. Knight swiftly examined Kiara's upper body. When he reached her abdomen, he slowed down. He gently examined her belly, starting at the top and moving down.

"Ouch, careful—that really hurts," Kiara protested, as Dr. Knight pressed down on the lower left part of her abdomen.

"The good news is that your appendix is on the other side," said Dr. Knight.

He leaned back and stuck his head out of the curtain. "Is there a nurse available? I'm ready for the pelvic," he called.

A woman came in, pulling a tray. "Okay, sweetie, go ahead and lie back. Is your friend staying?," the nurse asked.

"Yes," Kiara nodded, reaching for Madison's hand.

When Dr. Knight inserted the speculum, the pain intensified. The nurse handed him several swabs in succession, and Kiara let out her breath as he removed the instrument. But when he began to perform the second part of the exam, Kiara involuntarily cried out.

"That was your cervix, Kiara, the opening to your uterus. I'm sorry that hurt you, but it looks like you've got a pretty bad pelvic infection. I need to do a couple of lab tests and get an ultrasound of your belly."

"So you don't think it's appendicitis?," asked Madison.

"No. She's tender on her left, and the appendix is on the right."

"Then what do you think it is?," Madison pressed.

"Well, I need to make sure it's not an ectopic pregnancy," Dr. Knight replied. "That's also known as a tubal pregnancy. Basically it's when an early pregnancy happens in the fallopian tubes instead of in the uterus. That's dangerous because the tubes are not large enough to hold a growing embryo, so they can rupture and cause internal bleeding."

Kiara and Madison were silent, both remembering how their friend Lauren had needed to have surgery the year before for a tubal pregnancy.

"Kiara, the reaction you had when I did your exam strongly suggests that this is a pelvic infection. When someone has enough sudden sharp pain to cry out like you did when I examined your cervix, we call that a 'chandelier response,' meaning the pain is so severe that the patient jumps up toward the ceiling as though to grab a chandelier."

"As though there would ever be a chandelier in an exam room," smirked Madison.

"True," agreed Dr. Knight. "That expression is not meant to be funny though—simply descriptive of the intensity of the pain. At any rate, Kiara, the amount of pain you had during the exam is most consistent with a pelvic infection. Once we confirm it's not an ectopic pregnancy or an abscess, we should be able to treat you with antibiotics and let you go home."

"Can she get something for the pain?," asked Madison.

"Yes. I'm going to have the nurse start an IV, and we'll give her something to ease the pain and let her rest," answered Dr. Knight. He took Kiara's chart and slipped out between the curtains. The nurse cleaned up the tray and followed him while Dr. Knight instructed, "Here are her orders. I'm going to check on the chest pain in bed nine."

Madison held her friend's hand, trying to comfort her. "Don't worry, I'm sure they'll get you fixed up right away," she said. The two friends remained quiet, Kiara doubled in pain, and Madison listening to the bustling sounds of the ER outside their curtain-ringed cubicle. They waited for another fifteen minutes before anyone came back in to help Kiara. A short-haired brunette entered through the drapes, carrying a tray filled with tubes.

"Hi, I'm Brittany, and I'm here to draw your blood for a few tests."

"Are you starting her IV to give her some pain medicine too?," asked Madison.

"Nope, that's the nurse's job, but I did see Regina gathering supplies just now. Is she your nurse?," asked Brittany.

"We're not sure what her name is, but Kiara's nurse is wearing a scrub top with cats all over it, if that helps," answered Madison.

Brittany smiled. "That's definitely Regina. She loves all things cat. I'm sure she'll be right in." Brittany had already slipped a tourniquet around Kiara's arm and was drawing several tubes of blood. She swiftly finished her job, gently rolling Kiara back onto her side, where she stayed tucked in a fetal position. "All done," she announced brightly. "I'll check on your IV for you."

As she left, the drapes flapped open again, and Kiara and Madison looked up expectantly. The curtain was pulled all the way open, and a large cart was wheeled next to the exam table, pushed by a prematurely balding young man in navy scrubs.

"Hi, I'm Dave. Your doctor asked me to do an ultrasound of your abdomen and pelvis," he said, reaching down to plug his machine into an outlet in the wall behind the head of the exam table. "This might feel cold," he advised as he rolled Kiara onto her back, lifting her patient gown and squirting a clear gel on her belly. He pressed the transducer over Kiara's stomach with his right hand and adjusted the viewing screen with his left. Kiara bit her lip in discomfort.

"What are you looking for?," asked Madison.

"Well, this is the gallbladder over here, and I'll be looking at her liver, spleen, kidneys, bladder, ovaries, and uterus," Dave answered.

"Can you see the appendix?," asked Madison.

"Not well, but I can look for any abnormal swelling or fluid in that area," answered Dave, busy with his scan.

Regina stepped in with an IV bag, but retreated, saying, "Oops, sorry, Dave. I'll come back when you're done."

"Wait!," yelled Madison in vain, but the nurse had already left. "We've been waiting forever to get her some pain medicine," she explained to Dave, but he was too intent on his scan to respond.

Just when Kiara thought he must be finished, he began pressing hard on her left groin, making her squirm with pain. "Just hold still for a minute. If you can do that, I'll get done much faster. I know it hurts, but hang in there, okay? I'm hoping to avoid using the vaginal probe. You're thin enough that I might be able to get clear views from on top." That was plenty of information for Kiara. She struggled to remain as immobile as possible, willing to do anything to avoid any further internal exams. Dave made some adjustments on his machine and seemed to take a bunch of pictures and measurements too. "Okay, I'm done," he said at last.

"What did you see?," asked Madison, as Kiara turned back on her side and curled up.

"I only take the pictures, and it's up to the radiologist to read them. They really don't like me to say anything," he replied, gathering his equipment. "You should have the results in an hour or so."

"Things certainly don't move as fast here as they do on television, do they?" Madison tried to joke with Kiara. She peeked outside the curtain. "But seriously, I can see your nurse, and now for sure, you're getting that IV."

"Here I am," said Regina, brandishing an IV bag and supplies. Again, Kiara was moved onto her back. After a few minutes, the IV was running smoothly. "Okay, sweetie, now I can finally give you some medicine for pain," Regina said, reaching for a syringe. "You may get a funny taste in your mouth or feel burning in your arm, and then you'll feel sleepy."

"Thank you," whispered Kiara, rolling back on her side.

Nearly an hour later, Dr. Knight came back. "How's she doing?," he asked Madison.

"She's been asleep since they gave her the pain shot," answered Madison quietly. "But I think she's got a fever. She's been shaking some."

Dr. Knight looked at the chart. “Yes, her last temperature was 100.7 degrees. We’ll give her some Tylenol when she wakes up.”

“I’m awake,” slurred Kiara, rolling over and opening her eyes. “What did my tests show? What’s wrong?”

“As I suspected, you’ve got pelvic inflammatory disease, or PID for short,” Dr. Knight replied.

“What causes that?,” asked Kiara.

“PID comes from sexually transmitted infections, usually gonorrhea or chlamydia. Right now, I can’t tell you which one caused yours, but those test results should be available tomorrow. We will go ahead and treat you for both organisms, to cover all the bases. I also sent off tests for other STIs, including HIV, hepatitis C, and syphilis.”

“Because they cause PID too?,” asked Madison.

“No, because when you have one STI, you’re at risk for others. We’ll give you a prescription for an antibiotic that you’ll take by mouth to complete your treatment. You need to tell any sexual partners that they should be treated as well, or you can get reinfected easily.”

“There’s only one right now, and believe me, I’ll most certainly let him know,” fumed Kiara.

“Don’t forget Daniel, from last month,” added Madison.

“Thanks,” snipped Kiara, narrowing her eyes at her friend.

“I’ll have the nurse give you a handout on PID, but the main thing to know is that this is a serious infection, and you need to be certain you take all your medicine. This type of infection does put you at higher risk to develop a tubal pregnancy or infertility in the future.”

“Are you telling me I can’t have kids?,” asked Kiara incredulously.

“Not necessarily, but you do need to know that PID can cause permanent scarring and other problems in your reproductive organs, and while the antibiotics will cure the infection, they won’t cure any damage that has already happened.”

“So what’s the chance that I’ll be infertile?,” asked Kiara fearfully.

“Somewhere between one in five to one in eight women with a single case of PID become infertile,” advised Dr. Knight.

“But what about me? Do you think that I’ll be infertile from this? Can you tell? It seems like I’ve got a pretty bad case, from the pain I’m having,” Kiara agonized.

"I'm sorry, but there's no way to predict that," he answered.

"So how long should my pain last?"

"Usually that goes away within a few days of taking the antibiotics. Sometimes it can develop into chronic pelvic pain, and you should certainly follow up with your regular doctor if the pain lasts more than a week," he concluded.

"Are you going to give me something for the pain?"

"Of course, we'll give you some pain medication in addition to the antibiotics," the doctor reassured her.

"I've heard you should douche to clean out vaginal infections. Should Kiara do that?," asked Madison.

"I'm glad you asked that question," said Dr. Knight. "Absolutely do *not* douche. We think douching increases the risk of PID, likely by forcing what are often silent infections farther up the genital tract."

"So women shouldn't ever douche?," followed up Madison, pleased that Dr. Knight had finally appreciated her input.

"In my opinion, no. I would not recommend douching for any woman because we know it disturbs the normal balance of the flora in the vagina, and that can lead to bacterial vaginosis. Even worse, douching can spread a vaginal infection up higher into the reproductive organs. Douching is not only unnecessary, it's potentially harmful."

Both young women nodded their understanding.

"Let's make sure you get your full IV fluids and antibiotics, and then we'll let you check out. Your test results will be sent to you later this week. Here is a prescription for the oral antibiotic." He looked at Madison. "Can you help your friend get this filled tonight? I want to be sure she gets started on it as soon as possible. We'll give her the first dose before you leave." Dr. Knight turned back to Kiara. "I'd like you to follow up with your primary care physician. Do you have any more questions?"

Kiara had closed her eyes, this time to prevent tears. She was an only child and had long dreamed of raising a big family, with as many kids as she could stuff into an extra-large sport utility vehicle. The acting careers that she and Madison were pursuing were a fun diversion for now, but the only way theater fit into her long-term goals would be if she were directing a school play. "Focus on the positive," Kiara told herself, putting on her best performer's face.

"Only one. You said that basically I have, like, a four-out-of-five chance of this *not* impairing my future fertility, right?," Kiara rephrased with a positive spin.

Dr. Knight smiled. "Yes. As long as you don't get this again, that's correct." He paused for a second and then added, "Oh, and also assuming that when you were treated for chlamydia, it was discovered right away. The toughest part about STIs is that most of the time, people don't realize they have them."

"But the doctor said he cured my chlamydia infection back then!," retorted Kiara.

"Well, if you completed all the medicine he gave you, I'm sure it did cure that infection, but you can always get reinfected. There is no immunity, no future protection from having a past infection of either chlamydia or gonorrhea, and both diseases can be present without having any symptoms. The problem is that antibiotics treat the infection, but cannot repair any scarring that might have occurred in your reproductive system. Because your infection may have been silent, going untreated for some time, we don't know if there was any permanent damage. That's part of why it's so hard to make a prediction about your future fertility."

The doctor's words sank into Kiara as he turned to leave. Between the physical pain and fear of infertility, she barely heard his last comments. "I'll write your discharge orders now, but it will probably be another hour or so until your IV is done. A nurse will come unhook you and take care of all your paperwork at that time. Take good care of your friend," he directed Madison with a wink.

A few minutes passed while the two friends were immersed in their own thoughts, until Madison broke the silence. "Well, he's not exactly Dr. McDreamy, but I think he really warmed up to me at the end. Do you think he might be interested in me?," she asked hopefully.

All the acting classes in the world couldn't help Kiara mask her shock at her best friend's thought process. "That guy just did a pelvic exam on me. He told me I might not be able to have kids, and all you can think about is whether or not he's attracted to you?," she exploded. "I hardly think he's looking to date either of us."

"Hey, I'm not the one with an infection," Madison retorted defensively, instantly wishing she could take back the words as Kiara burst into tears.

"Oh, gosh, Kiara, I'm so sorry. I didn't mean it like that. It came out all wrong. I know it's not your fault. I'm sorry, and you're right. Everything's going to be okay," Madison babbled as she wrapped her friend in a hug. "You'll see, it will be all right," she murmured, holding her friend and wishing for the best.

9: Logan

LOGAN RAISED HIS ACHING head from the couch and surveyed the scores of empty beer bottles and several pizza boxes scattered all over the living room. Two people lay intertwined among blankets and pillows on the floor next to the couch where he had crashed. Spring break during his first year in law school was proving to be the wildest vacation of his life. Ten law school classmates had crammed themselves into a rented van and driven to Florida for its legendary beach parties. Hannah's dad owned this time-share right on the ocean, and their crowd filled the small luxury condo.

Logan carefully picked his way to the bathroom, stepping over sleeping bodies and trash along the way.

"Good morning, Logan," yawned a tall, curly-haired brunette dressed only in a T-shirt and underpants, as she headed into the bathroom ahead of Logan. "I'll be out in a second."

"Hey, Hannah," Logan muttered. A wave of nausea hit him, and Logan prayed he wouldn't start puking until he could get to the toilet. Luckily, Hannah was true to her word and came out in less than a minute. "All yours!"

"Thanks," breathed Logan, slipping past her into the bathroom, quickly closing the door and immediately reaching to grab the toilet seat. Logan seriously thought his head might explode as he retched repeatedly. "So not worth it," he thought repeatedly. "What the heck did we drink?"

Logan clearly remembered drinking beer all afternoon out on the beach. He vaguely remembered transitioning to the condo, but then everything was a complete blank. Never before in his life had he drunk so much that he couldn't remember stuff, but try as he might, his last clear memory was dancing out on the beach. The scruffy, pale guy staring back at him in the mirror offered nothing beyond the fact that he was still wearing the same swim trunks and T-shirt as yesterday. Logan was flustered: he physically felt like dirt and hated this sense of loss of control, not knowing exactly what had happened. He kept replaying his last memory, trying to force it to clear as he finished up in the bathroom. "What the... ?" He squinted downward. "Why is this burning so badly?" As Logan finished urinating, he noticed a white discharge at the tip of his penis.

Panic set in as Logan washed his hands. "Oh no! What did I catch? What the heck happened last night? Can you even get something this quickly?," he fretted. "If anyone finds out about this, I'll die of embarrassment. Maybe it will go away on its own," he hoped. "Of course, if it gets worse tomorrow, on the twenty-two-hour ride back to Texas, I'll be screwed." As he washed his hands, he looked at himself in the mirror, shaking his head. "Buck up, buddy. Go find a walk-in clinic and just get this fixed today." Logan wiped his hands dry and gingerly headed to the kitchen.

"Need a hangover omelette?," offered Hannah. "Here, start with this Gatorade and some crackers while I cook. No offense, but you look awful."

Logan cringed, but obediently sat on the barstool at the counter and started sipping his Gatorade. "Thanks, Hannah."

"Man, you were pounding it hard last night, Logan! I've never seen you like that. Since when do you do shots?"

"Since he had hot girls offering him belly shots," laughed J.R. as he walked up and reached fruitlessly for a high five from Logan.

"Yeah, right," growled Logan. "Whatever I had, it was so not worth it, I can tell you that much."

Pretty soon several other hungover revelers crawled up to the kitchen counter looking for food.

"I can't believe it's already Friday," moaned Jeff.

"I don't want to head back, but I think my liver needs detox," joked Lexie.

"My liver, my head, my stomach," added Sarah.

"Don't forget your sunburned skin," finished Maria.

"Let's hope we didn't do any permanent damage," laughed Jeff.

Logan discreetly knocked on the wooden counter in silent agreement.

"Just remember, what happens in Florida . . . ," started Sarah.

"Stays in Florida!," they chanted.

"Why do they have to be so dang loud?," Logan wondered irritably to himself. The chatter picked up as the food disappeared, and soon everyone was talking about their plans for the last day of spring break. Luckily for Logan, no one had claimed the car yet.

"Hey, Hannah, where did you put the car keys?," Logan asked. "I'll tell you what. I volunteer to go into town, put gas in the tank, and stock up on munchies for the ride back."

"No, Logan, you should relax and go back to sleep. I don't mind running into town. I have a list of things I want to pick up anyway. Thanks though," she said breezily.

Sarah joined in: "Hey, Hannah, I want to come too. I call shotgun."

"Not me," said Maria. "I'm headed back to the beach. I want to enjoy every last minute of this vacation."

Logan needed the car, and privacy. He tried to act like he felt much better than he did. "Honestly, your hangover eggs fixed me right up. I really don't mind running errands. I'd kind of like to drive around a bit and check out some of the town, since we've really only seen the beach. Text me whatever you guys want, and I'll get it, no problem. Since you got us this place, it's the least I can do," he practically pleaded.

Sarah gave in immediately. "Will you get me a candy bar? I'm having a serious craving for chocolate. I'll give you the money right now," she said, leaning to reach for her purse. "Come on, Hannah, let's go scope out the parties down the beach. You know there's going to be a ton of free stuff today since it's Friday, and I want to grab some T-shirts and baseball caps as souvenirs."

Hannah hesitated. "Logan, you're sure you don't mind?"

"Positively," said the relieved Logan. "You guys make a list of everything we need, and I'll take care of it."

A couple of hours later, Logan pulled into a parking lot under a sign advertising "Now Open: 24 Hour Medi-Quick Clinic." The odors of bleach and new carpet permeated the air, which didn't help his queasy stomach. "Well, it looks respectable," thought Logan hopefully. Before he had spied this clinic, he had passed by a few strip-mall doctors' offices that looked pretty sketchy.

"Good afternoon, how can I help you?," offered the receptionist.

"I'd like to see the doctor," responded Logan.

"Please fill out these forms and then bring them back to me along with your method of payment," said the receptionist.

"Thank you, ma'am," responded Logan politely, in his best courtroom voice. He sat down and began to fill out the forms. Logan was relieved that there were only two other people sitting in the waiting room. That meant he might get seen quickly.

"What a week," Logan reflected. "Who would've thought I'd end up here?" Surprises from the very first night they arrived in Florida had set a tone of decadence for the week. Exhausted from the long drive, the group had staggered into the condo around midnight, everyone lugging their backpacks or suitcases.

"Sarah and I claim the front bedroom with the ocean view and twin beds for the first night," declared Hannah. "Everyone feel free to fight over the rest," she added, tossing her luggage strap over her shoulder and disappearing into the hallway.

J.R. and Lexie had been snuggling in the van, so it was no surprise when they claimed the back room.

"I'm going to check out the beach scene, so don't wait up for me," said Jeff, dropping his stuff on the floor and appearing to catch a second wind.

"I'll join you," said Brandon, always up for a party.

Samantha looked around and said, "Okay, I'll crash with Logan here on the pullout couch."

Logan had assumed this was a purely platonic sleeping arrangement, until the lights went out. "Ever heard of friends with benefits?," whispered Samantha seductively, pressing her chest against Logan and moving one of her legs across his thighs.

"Seriously?," Logan replied, incredulously.

"Absolutely no strings attached. Let's get spring break started off right," she said, rubbing his chest.

"Why not?," wondered Logan, though he had never had casual sex before. Samantha's gorgeous green eyes and her ample chest had long tempted him, though her aggressive personality had kept him at bay. He let himself respond to her kisses and then disclosed, "I don't have any, uh, protection, with me, but I'm pretty sure Jeff does. Do you want me to go and get something?"

"No problem, I'm on the pill," Samantha replied.

The next morning, Logan woke up with second thoughts, worried about what Samantha might expect. Surprisingly, Samantha didn't act any differently with him than she had the entire year since they had met, and when she and Kristy brought two guys back to the condo the second night, Logan realized Samantha definitely wasn't looking for anything more from him.

After that, Logan had completely relaxed and partied along with his classmates. J.R. had ceremonially distributed a handful of condoms to the three other guys the first morning, encouraging them to practice safe sex. Logan was surprised to find himself needing one of them but thankful for the protection when he hooked up with a local waitress named Gabriela later in the week. She and her friends had joined their beach party last night too—though he still couldn't remember anything after drinking beers with them on the beach. Did he sleep with her again? Or worse, did he sleep with one of her friends? He realized that none of them were in the apartment when he woke up this morning. Logan involuntarily flushed, embarrassed by even a vague memory that he could be so...so out of control. Logan had always prided himself on being responsible, and he was happy to be the designated driver more often than not. He enjoyed his reputation of being that "good guy" that parents approved of for their daughters. And now, after a week of pure decadence that had seemed like such a harmless release from the intense rigor of law school, he was hungover and waiting to find out if he had a sexually transmitted infection.

"If I do have an STI, which girl gave me this?," he wondered, though he was pretty sure it was Samantha, because they hadn't used a condom.

"Logan?," said a young man in white scrubs from the doorway, interrupting Logan's thoughts.

"That's me," he answered.

"I'm Jaime, the medical assistant here," said the man. He weighed Logan, took him into an exam room, and charted all of Logan's vital signs. "So you've noticed a discharge?," he asked, reading the form Logan had filled out.

"Yes, just today," answered Logan.

"Any burning?"

"Only when I urinate," replied Logan evenly.

"Have you had unprotected sex with any new partners recently?"

Embarrassed, Logan limited his answer to a monosyllabic yes. In his mind, however, he added, "Which I know was incredibly stupid. I've been a decadent moron all week. In the heat of the moment, I simply didn't think." Admitting that he chose not to use a condom felt completely ignorant.

"Okay, the doctor will be in to examine you shortly," said Jaime. "Please get undressed from the waist down and have a seat on the exam table."

"Undressed? Can't I just pee in a cup or something?," inquired Logan.

"We can test for some bacterial STIs with urine samples, but Dr. Martinez still needs to examine you to be sure he's not missing anything else," replied the assistant.

Logan shrugged his assent, covered himself with the paper drape, and waited for the doctor.

About fifteen minutes later, the door popped open. "Hello, I'm Dr. Martinez," said a young man, impeccably dressed in pressed khakis, a white button-down shirt, and a festive tie, topped with a starched white lab coat. "Down here for spring break?"

"Yes," clipped Logan, not feeling particularly social.

The doctor perused his chart. "Looks like you might have had a bit too much fun," he commented. "When did you first notice any symptoms?"

"First thing when I urinated this morning," replied Logan.

"No fever, nausea, or rash?," asked the doctor.

"Well, nausea... but I assume that's from drinking last night. So,

I guess only the discharge and stinging," said Logan.

"Make sure you hydrate really well today with sports drinks for your hangover," said the doctor kindly. "If you are still nauseated now, we can easily give you some medicine to help with that, but you need the fluids to get rid of the headache I'm guessing you have as well. Meanwhile, let's take a look at you." Dr. Martinez set down the chart.

The doctor listened to Logan's heart and lungs, and then instructed Logan to lay back for the abdominal exam. When Dr. Martinez reached Logan's pubic area, he commented, "I definitely see the discharge you were talking about. You've also got some swollen lymph nodes here in your groin, which is expected, but I don't see anything else."

Logan's natural curiosity got the best of him, and he blurted, "What else would you see? I don't mean to be rude, but what else causes this symptom?"

Dr. Martinez grinned. "Honestly, it's less that I'm looking for a different cause for your discharge, and more that I'm making sure you don't have any additional infections. We see a lot of pubic lice, better known as crabs, as well as genital herpes and warts. Discharge can be associated with the viral infections too, though not typically this noticeable."

"Sorry I asked," groaned Logan.

"I'll run a couple of tests to confirm it, but it looks like you may have gonorrhea. There aren't too many infections where we see obvious discharge like this in guys. When was your contact with a new partner?"

"Sunday night," replied Logan and then, after a brief pause, he sheepishly added, "or possibly Wednesday night, but that time I used a condom. Um, and possibly last night."

Dr. Martinez raised an eyebrow but replied evenly, "Nothing would show up today from last night, but either of your other encounters could be the right timing. Of course, it's more likely from the time that you didn't wear a condom. When gonorrhea is symptomatic, it can appear as early as two days after exposure, although it can be as much as thirty days later." The doctor took a long, skinny package from his lab coat pocket. He opened it, removing a test tube and a swab. "This will sting a bit," he informed Logan. "We test for both gonorrhea and chlamydia, because those two diseases like to travel together."

He took a sample of the discharge from Logan's penis and then broke off the tip of the swab in the test tube and capped the tube. Then he removed another swab from a wrapper and took a second sample of the discharge. "I'll look at this one under the microscope right now," he said. "Go ahead and get dressed, and I'll be back in a couple of minutes."

Logan quickly pulled on his underwear and jeans, relieved to be dressed again. In a few minutes, Dr. Martinez returned.

"What I saw under the microscope was consistent with gonorrhea. There were a bunch of white blood cells, which shows inflammation. For a definitive test for chlamydia and gonorrhea, we send out to the lab."

"When will I get the results?," Logan asked.

"We should have them on Monday," replied the doctor.

"Monday?," Logan repeated, alarmed.

"Don't worry. I'll give you antibiotics today. The test is a confirmation, in this case primarily so you can inform your partners that they need to be treated. Actually, you should tell anyone you've had intimate contact with for at least the past month."

Logan felt foolish, but for some reason he didn't want the doctor to think he slept around indiscriminately. "Believe me, these two are it. I hadn't slept with anyone in over a year prior to this week."

"Busy week, then. Spring break can be dangerous," commented Dr. Martinez. "When you get back home, you need to go to your regular doctor and get tested for all STIs. I can do it here if you'd like, but usually people want to be sure their insurance will cover it, because it's pretty expensive."

"What else do you think I need to be tested for?," asked Logan.

"Blood tests are available for HIV, hepatitis C, syphilis, and herpes," answered Dr. Martinez.

"I can't imagine Samantha would have anything like that," Logan mused out loud, picturing his confident, assertive classmate.

"Think about it, Logan," said the doctor. "All STIs are basically passed the same way. If you have one, you're at risk for the others.

Don't kid yourself that 'nice girls,' or 'nice guys' for that matter, won't have bad diseases. Hopefully all you've caught is one or two bacterial illnesses, both of which we can cure."

"How are you going to treat me?," asked Logan.

"We're going to give you a shot of one antibiotic and a single dose of two pills of another. The shot will cover gonorrhea, and the pills will treat chlamydia."

"Is the shot penicillin? They say it cures everything, but I think I'm allergic to it," said Logan.

"Actually, about the only STI that penicillin still cures is syphilis. Everything else is resistant. The shot we're going to give you is ceftriaxone, which is a cousin of penicillin. In theory, there's about a ten percent chance of you also being allergic to it if you have a true penicillin allergy, but in practice we rarely see that. What was your symptom of allergy to penicillin?"

"I really don't know. My mom said I got a rash or something when I was little, and they thought it might be an allergic reaction to penicillin," said Logan.

"I think you'll be fine. Do you have any other questions for me?," asked the doctor.

Logan thought for a minute. He had tons of questions, though not all were for the doctor. "Knowledge is power," they say, so he'd better start arming himself. "How common is this? Is this what they call the clap?"

"Yes, 'the clap' traditionally refers to gonorrhea, and it is more common than you'd think. Chlamydia is the most common bacterial STI, with almost three million infections per year. Gonorrhea is the second most common one, at roughly seven hundred thousand new cases per year. Trichomoniasis is the most common nonviral STI overall, at over seven million new cases per year, but it doesn't usually cause a visible discharge," instructed Dr. Martinez.

"Once I take the antibiotic, then am I completely cured? Also, does this make me immune in the future?," Logan asked.

"Yes, you should be cured. I doubt you've had it long enough to cause permanent damage. Some cases can lead to infertility in men, but that's usually because guys are asymptomatic, not realizing they're carrying around a silent infection for years," the doctor explained. "However, you will not be immune to getting it again. These antibiotics will treat this infection, but you can catch it again."

"How often do girls know they have this disease?," asked Logan, wondering about Samantha.

"Somewhere between twenty and forty percent of women have no symptoms. It's important for them to be diagnosed so they don't develop scarring and other problems that lead to infertility. Obviously, you need to let your partners know that they should be treated," concluded Dr. Martinez.

"Can you just give me extra medicine to treat my, uh, partners? I mean, I know you wouldn't hand me a shot to give to someone, but are there pills available that would work just as well?," asked Logan.

"Not in Florida. I saw from your paperwork that you're in law school, so you might find this interesting. If I were to give you medicine to deliver to anyone you have been intimate with, that's called expedited partner therapy, or EPT for short. The original idea for EPT was that we would be more successful in cutting down on the spread of STIs if we made treatment more accessible that way. The downside is that we are treating a patient we've never seen, who could have underlying medical issues or drug allergies that could create a problem. Since 2006, thirteen states have prohibited EPT, and Florida is one of them. Texas, I believe, allows it under certain circumstances, but right now I'm afraid you're out of luck."

"I guess I feel badly about the second girl, in case I passed this on to her," Logan admitted.

"Send her over, and we'll take care of her," said Dr. Martinez cheerfully. "Anything else, or are you ready for your medicine?"

"One last question. I've been living in a three-bedroom condo with anywhere from ten to twenty people on a given night this week. How contagious is this? Could we have passed it to one another in the bathroom?"

"Only if you were having sex in there," Dr. Martinez replied with a chuckle. "These infections are not passed on toilet seats, despite popular myths. STIs are transmitted by intimate contact, either by genital-genital contact, oral-genital contact, genital-anal contact, or sharing sex toys. If you stayed clear of those, you're not guilty of putting your roommates at risk." Dr. Martinez stood up to leave. "My assistant, Jaime, will be back in with your medicines, and we'll contact you on Monday with your test results. Your symptoms should clear up quickly over the next couple of days. By the way, since this is likely your last night here, I should tell you that it's okay to drink alcohol with these antibiotics, but as a general principle, I'd limit it to a couple of drinks at the most. Good luck."

"I'm back to being the designated driver tonight, but thanks."

Jaime came in and smoothly delivered the shot, which stung like crazy, and watched while Logan swallowed two capsules. "Okay, you're free to check out," he instructed.

" 'Free' might not have been the most appropriate word," thought Logan. Back in the van, although several hundred dollars lighter, he breathed a sigh of relief. "At least I'm treated," he concluded. He glanced at his watch, which showed 2:30 p.m. "Okay, I've got time to get the groceries and gas, and I can slip into Dos Margaritas and find Gabriela." He knew she'd be upset, but if he left Florida without telling her, his conscience would never let him rest. Logan planned to spend his last night on the beach, simply enjoying the waves and rehydrating with more Gatorade. Alcohol and women were definitely not on his list tonight.

"How should I confront Samantha?," Logan wondered. "In fairness, Samantha may have no idea that she has this infection. Knowing her, I'd better wait 'til I have proof from the tests." In mock trials at school, Logan had seen Samantha rip apart arguments that lacked substance, and by no means did he want to face her unarmed. On the other hand, Logan realized there was a reasonable chance that on this, the last night of spring break, Samantha could become a repeat offender. "I'll actually be an accessory if I don't tell her today," he realized.

Logan started the van and headed out of the parking lot in search of the nearest grocery store. The debate persisted in his head, bringing in new factors. "What if she makes a huge scene and accuses me of giving this to her? What will everyone think? Who will they believe?" Samantha could be like a pit bull, never letting go once she got her teeth in something, and Logan had no desire to spend nearly twenty-four hours in a van listening to her hold forth.

"What if I hear she also slept with Jeff or J.R.? Should I tell them?" Logan's internal arguments continued until his legal intellect was exhausted. "I guess the jury's still out on this one," he conceded. "I don't know what I'm going to do."

facts

Gonorrhea Fact Sheet

What is it?

- Gonorrhea is a sexually transmittable infection caused by the *Neisseria gonorrhoeae* bacteria.

How common is it?

- The CDC reports that 333,004 people were infected in 2013 in the United States, though it should be noted that, because many infections are asymptomatic, it's likely that there were twice that many cases.

- In 2009, the United States reached a historic low number of cases, and there was renewed hope of eradicating gonorrhea, but antibiotic resistance and other factors have led to an increase in reported cases since 2009.

- Gonorrhea is the second most commonly reported bacterial sexually transmitted infection in the United States (behind chlamydia).

- 20- to 24-year-old women have the highest rate of gonorrhea at 541.6 cases per 100,000, which is more than 5 times the overall national average (106.1 per 100,000).

- For the first time since 2000, in 2013 the rate of reported cases was higher among men (109.5 per 100,000) than women (102.4 per 100,000).

- Significant racial disparity exists with gonorrhea; African Americans have much higher rates than Caucasians or Hispanics (426.6 per 100,000 vs. 34.5 and 65.8 per 100,000, respectively).

How do you get it?

- Gonorrhea is transmitted through oral, vaginal, penile, or anal sexual contact with an infected partner.

- Ejaculation does not need to occur to transmit the disease.

- Gonorrhea lives in semen and in vaginal secretions.

- It can be passed to a baby during vaginal childbirth.

Where on your body do you get it?

- Women usually get infections in the cervix or urinary tract.

- Men get infections in the urethra or epididymis.

- Eye, mouth, and anus infections can occur in either sex.

- Gonorrhea can spread to the blood or joints.

How do you know you have it?

- Many people are asymptomatic, so they only know they have gonorrhea if they choose to get tested.
- Men typically have penile discharge and burning with urination, and can also have painful swelling of the scrotum from epididymitis, which can lead to infertility.
- Women can have vaginal discharge, spotting between periods or after intercourse, pelvic pain, or painful urination.
- Both men and women can develop rectal symptoms, including itching, pain, discharge, bleeding, or pain with bowel movements.
- Tests are conducted from a urine sample or a sample of fluid from the cervix, penis, or throat, depending on the location of symptoms. There is no readily available blood test for gonorrhea.
- Pregnant women are routinely screened for gonorrhea.
- All sexually active women should be screened at their annual exam.
- Infertile couples may discover that past gonorrhea infections caused scarring of the woman's fallopian tubes.

What does it look like?

- Normal anatomy, or mild red irritation of the cervix, penis, or anus, with or without a white, yellow, green, or bloody discharge.

What does it feel like?

- Often, people are unaware that they have gonorrhea. An estimated 20%–40% of women and 10% of men have no symptoms.

- If symptoms are present, they include discharge (penile or vaginal) and burning with urination.

- Women can notice vaginal bleeding between periods.

- Advanced infection can cause pelvic inflammatory disease (PID), which causes intense pelvic and abdominal pain, vaginal bleeding, vomiting, or fever.

- Rectal disease produces discharge, itching, soreness, bleeding, or painful bowel movements, or may be asymptomatic.

- Testicular pain comes from epididymitis.

How long does it last?

- Gonorrhea infections can exist silently for an unknown period of time until treated.

- Active symptoms can appear in two days to several weeks after exposure.

- Symptoms usually resolve quickly with antibiotic treatment, unless there is antibiotic resistance.

Can it be cured?

- Yes. Antibiotics can completely eliminate the bacteria, although they will not reverse any damage done by gonorrhea (such as scarring of the fallopian tubes or epididymis). However, there is a great deal of antibiotic resistance, especially in Asia and the United States, with more developing each year. This means that gonorrhea is becoming more difficult to treat as it becomes resistant to standard antibiotic therapy.

Can you be reinfected?

- Yes. Prior episodes of gonorrhea infection offer no protection. Reinfection is very common, especially when a partner is not fully treated.
- Each subsequent infection with gonorrhea significantly increases the risk of long-term consequences.

What is the treatment?

- Steadily increasing antibiotic resistance has created an enormous challenge in treating gonorrheal infections. Antibiotics recommended to treat gonorrhea in the past included ceftriaxone, cefixime, ciprofloxacin, ofloxacin, and levofloxacin, usually in a single dose. As of April 2007, the CDC changed its guidelines, no longer recommending any of the fluoroquinolones listed above (ciprofloxacin, ofloxacin, and levofloxacin) due to the advanced drug resistance of gonorrhea.
- The CDC recommends testing or directly treating for chlamydia at the same time (with different antibiotics) because the two diseases are commonly present together.
- Notify anyone you have had sexual contact with in the last two months, so their doctors can treat them for gonorrhea regardless of whether or not they have symptoms.

How about alternative therapies?

- None are proven to eliminate gonorrhea.

Are there long-term consequences?

- Estimates vary, but 10%–30% of untreated gonorrhea infections in women will go on to cause pelvic inflammatory disease (PID). Gonorrhea and chlamydia are the primary causes of all PID.

- PID causes scarring and blockage of fallopian tubes, causing an estimated 100,000 women annually to become infertile.

- PID scarring can also cause ectopic or tubal pregnancies (pregnancies occurring outside the uterus), which are potentially life threatening.

- PID can lead to chronic pelvic pain.

- Newborns exposed to gonorrhea through the birth canal can develop throat infections or serious eye infections leading to blindness if not treated in the first few weeks of life.

When are you contagious?

- Any time you are infected with gonorrhea, regardless of symptoms.

- Even while using a condom. Latex male condoms can greatly reduce but not completely eliminate transmission of gonorrhea from an infected male to his partner.

Can gonorrhea be transmitted between homosexual partners?

- Male homosexual transmission occurs via anal and oral sex.

- Female-to-female genital transmission is theoretically possible but not proven.

How do I avoid getting gonorrhea?

- Abstaining from oral, vaginal, and anal sex is 100% effective.
- Consistent and correct use of condoms will dramatically reduce the risk for transmission of gonorrhea from a male to his partner, as long as the condom does not break.
- Use new condoms for each partner with any shared sex toys or, preferably, do not share sex toys.
- Female barrier methods and spermicides are less effective than condoms but do decrease transmission somewhat.
- Have intercourse only within a monogamous relationship in which both partners have tested negative for gonorrhea.

If I have gonorrhea, how do I avoid giving it to my partner?

- If you have had no sexual contact yet with your partner, abstain from oral, vaginal, and anal sex until you complete your antibiotics and any symptoms have resolved.
- If there has been any prior sexual contact with your partner, abstain from oral, vaginal, and anal sex until both of you have completed antibiotic therapy and any symptoms have resolved.

Frequently Asked Questions

➤ **Is gonorrhea the same as chlamydia? Aren't they both "the clap"?**
No. "The clap" typically refers to gonorrhea. The symptoms of both diseases are often identical, but different bacteria cause chlamydia and gonorrhea, so they require treatment with different antibiotics.

➤ **Will penicillin cure gonorrhea?**
No. Currently, the only class of antibiotics recommended to reliably kill gonorrhea is the cephalosporin class, which is a cousin of penicillin.

➤ **Can you get gonorrhea from a toilet seat?**
No.

➤ **Can you have chlamydia and gonorrhea at the same time?**
Yes, this happens commonly. If you have one, you should be tested and/or treated for the other one.

➤ **Can you get gonorrhea from douching?**
No. However, douching can cause pelvic inflammatory disease (PID) by forcing vaginal infections (often silent) up into the cervix and into the uterus or fallopian tubes.

Additional Information

American College of Obstetricians and Gynecologists
PO Box 70620
Washington, DC 20024-9998
1-800-673-8444
www.acog.org/publications/patient_education/bp071.cfm

American Sexual Health Association
PO Box 13827
Research Triangle Park, NC 27709
919-361-8400
www.ashasexualhealth.org/

Centers for Disease Control and Prevention
1600 Clifton Road
Atlanta, GA 30329-4027
1-800-CDC-INFO (1-800-232-4636), 1-888-232-6348 (TTY)
www.cdc.gov/STI/Gonorrhea/default.htm

MedlinePlus
US National Library of Medicine
8600 Rockville Pike
Bethesda, MD 20894
1-888-FIND-NLM (1-888-346-3656) or 301-594-5983
www.nlm.nih.gov/medlineplus/gonorrhea.html

DATE RAPE

10: Ashley

ASHLEY'S HEAD WAS POUNDING and her stomach was rolling. She forced her eyes open and immediately panicked. Where was she? Clearly this was a guy's room. Frat house or dorm?

"Oh, man, what did I drink last night? What did I do?" Her heart was racing as she clutched the sheet to her chest and tried to piece everything together. "I've got to get out of here. Crap, where are my clothes?" The panic rose as she realized she was only wearing the sheets. Ashley sat up quickly and almost fell back again as everything went black for a few seconds—and then the nausea exploded. Dragging the sheets with her, she lunged for the bathroom and began vomiting into the toilet. The only bright spot was that she found her clothes piled on the floor. She had never been so miserable and so terrified. Getting dressed between waves of puking, she eventually located her phone and wallet and stealthily crept out of the frat house. Sobbing, she texted her best friend, Olivia, and begged for help getting back to her dorm.

Olivia freaked out when Ashley dropped herself into the passenger seat. "Oh my gosh, what on earth happened to you? You look awful. You are so not a partier!," Olivia exclaimed.

"I'm really not," Ashley moaned. "You know me, I hold on to one cup of beer and pretend to drink it all night so no one will hassle me."

"I know, I know," reassured Olivia. "So what happened? The last time I saw you last night, it was really early and you said you were leaving, so I thought you had gone home, not over to another party. You definitely didn't seem drunk..."

Ashley started crying again, barely able to speak. The truth was, although she remembered telling Olivia goodbye, she didn't recall much else, and she definitely did not remember going to a frat house. She vaguely recalled some guys laughing when they gave her the sparkling water she had asked for, but everything was blank after that. Olivia quickly got Ashley back to their dorm and set out some Gatorade and crackers next to Ashley's bed, encouraging Ashley to "sleep it off" and "stay hydrated." Ashley thankfully crawled into her bed and spent the rest of the day trying to recover.

What followed was a horrible week. When the weekend arrived, Ashley had zero intention of heading to any parties after last Saturday's nightmare. Ashley not only felt physically lousy for a couple of days after she vomited so much, but rumors were making their way back to her that she had hooked up with a rugby player from her economics class. While she was not a virgin, Ashley had only been intimate with her high school boyfriend, and Colton was two states and five hours away at another university. And yet, there was no denying the fact that she had woken up naked in a guy's room on Sunday morning. Her heart raced as she remembered her terror that morning. She didn't feel as though she had been raped—she had no bruising or soreness—but could she have had sex? Was it possible she somehow was so drunk that she voluntarily hooked up with someone? It was frightening to have no memory of that night, and specifically she had no memory of taking her clothes off. Or memory of who, if anyone, she was with. She shook her head in disbelief. No, surely she had not had sex. She would know. Wouldn't she? And on top of all the confusion and fear, she now had a sore throat that kept getting worse. Ashley decided she should make an appointment at the health center and check to be sure she wasn't coming down with strep throat or the flu or something. She pulled out her phone, found the website, and signed up for an urgent care spot the next morning.

Ashley woke up with her throat extremely uncomfortable, and she was thankful she had made the appointment. She wanted to take some Tylenol or Advil, but decided not to, in case they wanted to see if she had a fever. Her whole body ached as she hiked across campus to the health center. She checked in at the computer stand and was pleasantly surprised when she waited less than fifteen minutes before the medical assistant called her name and efficiently took her into an exam room, only stopping to get her weight along the way.

"It's official: you have a fever of 100.7 degrees," the assistant noted sympathetically as she put away the thermometer. "And your pulse is 108, which is probably from that temperature. The doctor will be in shortly to take a look at you."

Ashley pulled out her phone and automatically started mindlessly playing games. After a while, she got bored with that and wondered what was taking so long. Looking around the room, she started reading the posters. "Study Natural" featured an apparently naked co-ed peeking through library shelves and explained the risks of stimulant abuse. "Catch Some ZZZs" offered tips about sleep hygiene. But it was the next poster that grabbed her full attention.

THIS GIRL . . .
. . . cannot remember anything about last night
. . . only had one drink
. . . never thought it would happen to her

The poster promoted awareness about date-rape drugs. "Oh no! I didn't even think about whether I could have been drugged!," Ashley realized in a flash. She had been so busy blaming herself for drinking that it had not occurred to her that someone might have slipped something into her drink. Just as Ashley was processing this thought, the door opened and the doctor stepped in.

"Hi, Ashley, I'm Dr. Belk," said the young woman, sitting down on her rolling stool and logging onto the computer. "Sorry you are not feeling well. I understand you have a sore throat?"

"Yes," nodded Ashley.

"When did it start hurting?," asked the doctor.

"It started a day or two ago, but this morning it is really sore, and now I have a fever too," Ashley noted.

"Have you been having any allergy symptoms, like itchy eyes, runny nose, or sneezing?"

"No," Ashley answered.

"Any cough?"

"Not yet."

"That's optimistic." Dr. Belk smiled. "How about headache, body aches, or joint pains?"

"I am starting to feel achy everywhere, but no joint pains, and not really any headache," Ashley replied.

"Any stomach issues, like nausea, vomiting, or diarrhea?," asked the doctor.

"No," Ashley answered immediately, but then, "Well, not since last weekend..."

"Were you sick?"

"Well... it's embarrassing, but I... I think I drank too much at a party. I am really not a drinker at all, which is what makes it weird. But I woke up on Sunday morning and I was so sick that I vomited a ton, and I felt horrible all of Sunday and most of Monday too," Ashley admitted.

"So, how much did you drink? Or do you not remember?," asked Dr. Belk.

Ashley bit her lip as she felt tears welling up. "I really didn't come in to talk about that. I just have a bad sore throat and want to be sure it's not strep."

Dr. Belk gently smiled. "Ashley, I'm not judging you at all, but I do want to ask you more questions so I have a full picture medically, okay?"

Ashley nodded.

"So, let's go back to before last weekend. At that point, you were feeling totally healthy? No allergy symptoms, fevers, fatigue, anything?," she asked.

"No, I was totally fine."

"Then, I suppose, Saturday night you went to a party?," Dr. Belk inquired.

"Yes. Some of my friends and I went to a frat party. I usually have one or at the most two beers in an entire night. I'm the only one in my group that never does shots. But the last clear thing I remember about that night was walking into that party..." Her voice trailed off.

"Have you ever had a memory gap like this before?," inquired the doctor.

"Never! I've never even thrown up before," Ashley insisted. "I swear, the most alcohol I have ever had in one night was three drinks, and that was beer."

"And what do you remember next, after walking into the party?"

Ashley looked down and swallowed painfully. "I woke up in a different place. I was in another frat house, but no one else was in the room. I was so sick that I vomited four or five times, and I kept feeling like I was going to pass out. I was half relieved and half scared that no one else was around. When I finally stopped puking, a friend picked me up and took me back to my dorm."

"That must have been frightening for you," offered Dr. Belk.

"Extremely."

"Did you have any concern about whether you may have been taken advantage of sexually? Any pain or discomfort or signs of a struggle?," asked the doctor.

Ashley shook her head no. "I was nauseated and lightheaded and I felt awful, but I didn't feel violated in that way... I don't think."

"Were you still dressed?," asked Dr. Belk.

"Y-yes," lied Ashley, knowing she was flushing but feeling she could not tell this doctor any more details.

Dr. Belk sensed Ashley's unease and shifted gears. "What have your friends told you? Did any of them see you looking intoxicated that night?"

"No, it's so frustrating, because it's all a blank. My friends saw me holding my usual plastic cup of beer at the first party. Unfortunately, they all thought I went home, but apparently instead I went to a different frat house. None of my friends seem to have seen me leave, and no one has been willing to say anything directly to me if they saw me at the second place, where I woke up the next morning. To be fully honest, I know that people have been saying I hooked up with a guy at that second place. But if I did, I have zero memory of it, and I haven't had the nerve to ask that guy directly," she finished rapidly.

"Have you been sexually active in the past?," asked Dr. Belk.

"Yes. I'm on the pill, but I have only had one partner, my boyfriend, Colton. He goes to Georgia Tech though, so I haven't seen him in over a month."

"Okay. I'm sorry you didn't come in on Sunday, because at that point we could have done a drug screen on you to see if someone slipped you something, but now any of those drugs would be out of your system," explained Dr. Belk. "Not to mention, you probably could have used some IV fluids to rehydrate you and help you feel better. I am so sorry you had this experience. I encourage you to talk with one of our counselors today when we are done. Also, to be safe, I would recommend getting tested for STIs. We can take care of that today too."

"But can you please test me for strep also?," asked Ashley. "My throat hurts so much, and I have had strep a bunch in the past."

"Of course. Let's get through the rest of your history, and then I will take a look at you and perform a rapid strep test since you do have a fever, a sore throat, and no cough."

Dr. Belk ran through the rest of Ashley's medical history, taking notes on the computer. During her examination, Dr. Belk observed that Ashley's tonsils were very red and had pus on them and that her neck glands were swollen and tender. With a swab, she deftly reached back into Ashley's throat and got a sample to test. "Okay, we'll have the rapid strep back in around ten minutes, and then I can make a better decision on how to treat you," Dr. Belk said. "Meanwhile, I'll have my nurse come in and bring you a special numbing medicine to gargle to help your throat feel better."

By the time the nurse had given Ashley the medicine, which wonderfully numbed her throat, Dr. Belk was back in the room.

"Ashley, your rapid strep test was negative, so we do not have a definite cause of your sore throat yet," announced the doctor. "But with your swollen glands and fever along with your tonsils being so red and having pus, I want to be sure we are not missing anything else, like possibly mono. You've never had that before, right?"

"No, I haven't had mono to the best of my knowledge. My roommate had it last semester though," said Ashley.

"I'm going to have the medical assistant come and draw your blood to do a blood count and to look for mono, and I'm going to send off a throat culture to be sure the rapid strep didn't miss anything. To cover all our bases, I will also swab your throat for STIs, because they would require a different antibiotic. Meanwhile, I'm going to give you a prescription for some tetracaine lollipops, which will numb your throat in the same way that the gargle did. Do you want to use our pharmacy or one off-campus?," asked Dr. Belk.

"Um... the pharmacy here is fine, but what did you mean about checking for STIs in my throat? Can you actually get that kind of infection in your mouth?" Ashley grimaced.

"Absolutely. All of the sexually transmitted infections—except one called trichomoniasis—can be passed via oral sex. Herpes, for example, is very commonly passed from mouths to genitals, and less commonly vice versa—not that your throat looks like herpes. We also see gonorrheal infections in the throat sometimes. With the timing of this infection after your experience last weekend, I think it's prudent to check. Does that make sense?," asked the doctor.

Eyes wide, Ashley nodded. "So are you giving me an antibiotic?"

"Not at this point, because your strep test was negative. If you have mono or another viral illness, antibiotics won't help at all. We'll know more when we get the next set of results tomorrow, and we'll send you a secure message to let you know, okay?"

"Sure," Ashley agreed.

"Let me give you this too. It's good information about both alcohol poisoning and so-called date-rape drugs. At this point, there is no way for us to know what happened to you, but I want to be sure you have good resources to learn more. Our Teal Ribbon twenty-four-hour hotline number is on there too. They are there to answer any concerns about possible sexual assault. May I have one of the counselors come and visit with you before you leave?," offered Dr. Belk, as she handed Ashley a pamphlet.

Ashley took the brochure but declined the offer of a counselor. "Thank you, but I really don't feel well now, and I just want to get my prescription and go back to my dorm and rest. And I really don't think I was assaulted. I still think I may have strep throat."

"I understand. We'll contact you tomorrow with the rest of your results," said the doctor.

Ashley woke up the next morning feeling slightly better, which was encouraging. After her first class, she saw that she had a message from the health center, and she logged in to check her results.

> Dear Ashley,
>
> Your blood count and mono test did not show any signs of mononucleosis infection. Unfortunately, however, your throat swab was positive for gonorrhea. Please schedule an appointment today in urgent care so you can be treated with the appropriate shot of antibiotics. We have openings at 10:50 a.m., 11:20 a.m., and 3:30 p.m. Let us know what works best with your schedule. I will be available to answer any additional questions that you might have when you come in.
>
> Sincerely,
> Dr. Belk

Ashley's mouth dropped open in shock—and disgust. "I have gonorrhea in my throat? Are you kidding me?" Ashley involuntarily gagged at the thought. "And my friend Sabrina, who goes down on every guy she meets, has never caught a thing? This is so unfair!"

Ashley glanced at the time and started walking as fast as she could to the health center, responding to the secure message as she walked and claiming the first opening at 10:50 a.m., which was in less than ten minutes. She was trembling and felt like she was on the verge of losing control. "Please let that counselor be available today. I will definitely talk with her now," she thought.

Very quickly Ashley was back in the same exam room as the day before. The assistant took her vital signs and assured her that the doctor would be right in. Ashley stared again at the "THIS GIRL" poster, shaking her head in disbelief. "I am 'this girl,'" her thoughts echoed.

Dr. Belk stepped in the room and sat down. "Ashley, thank you for coming in so quickly. We are going to give you a shot of ceftriaxone, which is a cousin of penicillin, to cure your throat infection from gonorrhea. We will also follow the CDC guidelines and give you an oral antibiotic, azithromycin, in a single dose, which will completely cover you for a possible secondary infection with chlamydia. These antibiotics treat gonorrhea and chlamydia in any location on your body. I know you said you didn't believe you had been sexually assaulted, but obviously this is a sexually transmittable infection in your throat."

Ashley mumbled her agreement, or at least indicated that she was following what the doctor was saying, "Mm, hmm."

"I can't imagine how frightening this is for you, since you don't have any memory of that night. I really hope you will talk with one of our counselors today. They help students every day who have had similar experiences, and I think you will find they are not only compassionate, but very knowledgeable about the medical, emotional, and legal aspects of your situation. Meanwhile, I want to encourage you to have an HIV and syphilis test, so we can complete your STI screen."

"Oh my gosh, do you think I have HIV?," gasped Ashley.

"No, no. But any time someone has contracted or been exposed to one STI, they are obviously potentially at risk for any STI, so we recommend full testing," explained Dr. Belk. "Do you have any other questions for me?"

"I'm not sure." Ashley paused. "I guess I just want to be certain that this shot and the other medicine you're giving me will definitely clear up anything I might have caught. Is that correct?"

"The shot and pills will cure gonorrhea and chlamydia in your throat and anywhere else in your body," reiterated the doctor. "The viral sexually transmitted infections include HIV, HPV, and herpes, and while I have no indication that you are infected with any of these, I do want to be clear that they are not treatable with antibiotics."

Ashley nodded, gripping her crossed arms tightly as the doctor continued.

"Additionally, since people are understandably most concerned about HIV, please know that it is too early after your potential exposure last week for an HIV test to indicate a positive result. We will repeat your blood tests for both HIV and syphilis in six weeks, three months, and six months. Testing you today for HIV will hopefully confirm for us that you were not previously infected. You mentioned yesterday that you are sexually active with a long-term boyfriend. Have you both been tested for STIs?"

"No, because we were both virgins when we got together," replied Ashley.

"And do you use condoms?"

"Again, no, because I'm on the pill, and we weren't worried about STIs," answered Ashley.

"For the future, I would encourage you to always use condoms, both as extra protection for birth control and as a barrier protection against STIs—even for oral sex," noted Dr. Belk. "And of course, you should encourage your boyfriend to get tested."

"Frankly, I don't want to have any kind of sex in the near future," Ashley sobbed. Dr. Belk stood up and nodded to the nurse. "Let's get you treated now, and I will ask the counselor to come and talk with you to answer any further questions you might have."

Ashley clenched her jaw and nodded. She had a ton of questions. Perhaps not as many for the counselor as for her friends and for that rugby guy. And for herself. What would she tell her boyfriend? *Would* she tell him?

facts

Date Rape Fact Sheet

What is date rape?

- Date rape refers to nonconsensual sexual intimacy (including oral, anal, or vaginal intercourse) between two people who know each other.
- Sexual assault and rape are frighteningly common in the United States—nearly 1 in 5 women and 1 in 71 men are rape victims at some point in their life, and over half of the assaults on women are by an "intimate partner."
- College campuses report 1 in 4 female students and 1 in 7 male students are victims of sexual assault; 85% of rapes on campus are date rapes.
- Only a small fraction (perhaps as low as 5%) of rapes are reported to authorities.

- Approximately 75% of women victims whose sexual assault meets the legal criteria for rape do not believe themselves to have been raped.

- Date rape is a felony, the same as rape committed by a stranger.

What are date-rape drugs?

- "Date-rape drugs" typically refer to sedative drugs in the benzodiazepine class (such as the brand name drugs Valium, Xanax, and Rohypnol), GHB (gamma-hydroxybutyrate, a synthetic neurotransmitter), and Ketamine (an anesthetic), which are slipped into drinks without the person's knowledge and with the intent of lowering the person's inhibitions and making sexual assault easier.

- Alcohol alone is the most common agent used for this purpose.

- The combination of alcohol and sedatives is very dangerous, augmenting the actions of both drugs to cause sedation, impaired judgment, confusion, and memory loss.

- GHB (gamma-hydroxybutyrate) is the most commonly used date-rape drug, with street names that include Georgia Home Boy, Liquid Ecstasy, Easy Lay, Cherry Meth, Liquid X, Scoop, Salt Water Soap, and G-Caps.

- GHB was originally developed as an anesthetic, but it has been used over the years as a nutritional supplement and sleep aid. The FDA banned the use of GHB in 1990 because seizures, hospitalizations, and deaths were related to these products, but people still obtain GHB over the Internet or in health food stores.

- GHB is an odorless, colorless, salty-tasting liquid or powder that can easily be slipped into drinks.

- The drug produces an immediate sense of euphoria, followed very rapidly by confusion and agitation. The person blacks out within fifteen minutes and has a significant risk of seizures.

- There is no way to reverse the effects of GHB; the only treatment is supportive.

- Rohypnol (flunitrazepam) is also known as Roofies, Circles, Mexican Valium, and R-2.

- Flunitrazepam is banned in the United States but is frequently smuggled in from Latin America, where it is a legal drug used during surgery or to treat insomnia.

- Flunitrazepam is an odorless, tasteless, oblong, 1 mg or 2 mg (hence, "R-2"), olive-green tablet with the number 542 imprinted on top.

- The manufacturer has now added a dye to the tablet, which should make a clear drink turn blue (dark drinks such as cola should turn cloudy), to help increase awareness of illicit use.

- Flunitrazepam is often used voluntarily as a recreational drug because of its rapid effects of euphoria and loss of inhibition.

- Confusion and memory loss (which may include memory loss of the brief time before the person consumed the drug, as well as the time of intoxication) appear to variable degrees after the initial effects. These symptoms are magnified when the drug is combined with alcohol, which is typically the case.

- The effects of flunitrazepam can be medically reversed by another drug: flumazenil.

- Ketamine is the third most commonly used date-rape drug.

- Ketamine is known on the street as Kit-Kat, Special K, Cat Valium, Jet, Black Hole, Purple, and Super Acid.

- Ketamine is a dissociative anesthetic, meaning that it causes hallucinations and distortions of the senses (especially vision and hearing), including a feeling of detachment from the body in a dreamlike state.

- Ketamine also may cause amnesia (memory loss), nausea, or vomiting.

- Ketamine is produced as a liquid or as a white powder that easily dissolves in liquid.

- Ketamine wears off very quickly, but the memory loss or distortion of the events for the time surrounding the intoxication typically persists.

How common is date rape?

- Sadly, one in four undergraduate women are estimated to be victims of sexual assault, and the majority of the assaults involve alcohol and/or drugs.

- The date-rape drugs are particularly frightening because the victim is not aware that he or she consumed anything extra, and the effects are immediate and intense, and usually include significant or complete memory loss or blackout periods.

- Compounding the issue is that often the victims are voluntarily drinking alcohol, and they believe that the assault was a result of their own conscious choices.

What should you do if you believe you were drugged?

- If you have the presence of mind during an acute intoxication to recognize that you have possibly just been drugged (because you are suddenly very "drunk" out of proportion to your consumption), immediately tell a trusted friend and ask that they take you directly for medical attention.

- More commonly, victims awake the next morning feeling "hungover" out of proportion to their consumption, with their clothes disturbed or other physical signs or symptoms that they have been sexually violated. If this happens, immediately go to the hospital, preferably taken there by a trusted friend. If you do not feel comfortable asking a friend, you can call a rape crisis hotline. These crisis lines are an excellent resource of information, compassion, and practical advice, and they can direct you (or accompany you) to a local provider where you can be examined and counseled. Do not shower, brush your teeth, change clothes, or even urinate (if you can wait) before you get to the hospital, because you have the perpetrator's DNA on you, which can be collected for up to 96 hours after the assault if not washed away.

What should you expect from sexual assault services at the hospital?

- Sexual assault nurse examiners are compassionate, trained professionals who will be taking care of you.

- Having evidence collected does not obligate you to press charges. You can make that decision later.

- First, you will sign a consent form. Next, you will tell the examiner your regular medical history, including any medications you take regularly, any surgeries, medication allergies, and so on. Then, you will be asked to tell the examiner everything you remember about the assault, understanding that you may know very little.

- Your clothing will be completely removed and kept as evidence (you will be given a patient gown or other clothing).

- Your examiner will take samples from your mouth, fingernails, and hair, and then she will do a genital exam.
- Blood and urine samples will be taken.
- You will then be able to clean up and get dressed (in different clothing from the clothes you arrived in), and the counselors will talk with you.
- You will be offered a chance to speak with law enforcement, if you choose.

How much will it cost to have an exam?

- The Violence Against Women Act (VAWA) of 1994, reauthorized on March 19, 2013, says that states must provide a free forensic medical exam directly, or provide reimbursement for such an exam, regardless of whether or not the victim chooses to press charges.
- Specific costs vary depending on your location and, possibly, your insurance.

How can I prevent getting drugged?

- Always get your own drink, or insist on opening a bottle yourself.
- Never set your drink down, and if you do, get a new drink.
- Always have a designated nondrinking friend in your group.
- If a drink tastes odd (especially if salty), pour it out.
- Recognize that if you are drinking alcohol, your alertness and judgment are already impaired.

How about alternative prevention?

- In 2014, students from North Carolina State University developed a nail polish called "Undercover Colors" that changes color if the finger is dipped into a drink that contains Rohypnol, Xanax, or GHB. Rape crisis centers, however, do not endorse this product because they feel that it reinforces the misconception that the prevention of sexual assault is the responsibility of the victim.

What STIs are tested for after sexual assault?

- Sexual assault exams test for gonorrhea, chlamydia, trichomoniasis, HIV, hepatitis B (unless the victim is immunized), and syphilis.

- Repeat testing is offered 1–2 weeks after the assault because not all STIs will test positive immediately.

- If initial tests are negative, additional testing for syphilis and HIV may be repeated at 6 weeks, 3 months, and 6 months after the assault.

What preventive treatment is offered after sexual assault?

- If the person has not received the hepatitis B immunization, then the hepatitis B vaccine series is initiated.

- Antibiotics may be given to treat potential chlamydia, gonorrhea, and trichomoniasis infections.

- Emergency contraception is offered if the victim could potentially become pregnant from the assault.

Frequently Asked Questions

➤ **How quickly do date-rape drugs start working?**
These drugs take effect very quickly, most of them within fifteen minutes.

➤ **If you have memory loss, does that prove you were drugged?**
No. Alcohol alone can cause memory loss. However, if your designated nondrinking trusted companion is certain you only had one or two drinks (of beer or wine, or a single shot of liquor) and you have significant memory loss, the odds are higher that you may have been drugged.

➤ **If you go to the hospital for an exam because you believe you have been assaulted, do you have to press charges?**
No, absolutely not. It's important to have an exam as soon as possible to collect evidence, because the longer you wait to do so, the lower the yield of evidence, but you do not need to decide about pressing charges at that time.

➤ **How often does sexual assault cause the victim to get an STI?**
Many sexual assaults go unreported, so the statistics are challenging to interpret, but it is estimated that 15% of sexual assaults result in STI transmission, often with more than a single type of infection.

➤ **What STIs are most commonly transmitted in cases of sexual assault?**
According to the CDC's 2011 statistics, gonorrhea, chlamydia, and trichomoniasis are the most common STIs diagnosed after sexual assault.

Additional Information

Factsheet: The Violence Against Women Act
www.whitehouse.gov/sites/default/files/docs/vawa_factsheet.pdf

A National Protocol for Sexual Assault Medical Forensic Examinations Adults/Adolescents (2nd ed., April 2013)
www.ncjrs.gov/pdffiles1/ovw/241903.pdf

National Sexual Assault Telephone Hotline
1-800-656-HOPE (1-800-656-4673)
www.rainn.org/get-help/national-sexual-assault-hotline

Office of National Drug Control Policy
www.whitehousedrugpolicy.gov

Rape, Abuse, and Incest National Network (RAINN)
1-800-656-HOPE (1-800-656-4673)
www.rainn.org

Rape Prevention and Education (RPE) Program
www.cdc.gov/ViolencePrevention/RPE/index.html

Undercover Colors
www.undercovercolors.com

Violence Against Women Reauthorization Act of 2013
www.govtrack.us/congress/bills/113/s47/text

TRICHOMONIASIS

II: Alyssa

SWEAT DRIPPED DOWN ALYSSA'S back as she jogged toward the final turn at Town Lake. "With weather this nice, I know I can stay motivated to keep exercising and lose these 'freshman fifteen' pounds I put on last year," she thought. Too many pizzas and beers, plus her love of Mexican food, had piled on the calories. Who can resist chips and queso? Not Alyssa, especially last semester when she was nursing a broken heart. "No sense in dwelling on the past," Alyssa chastised herself. She pushed herself into a sprint for the last half mile, clearing her mind of negative thoughts and visualizing her healthier body.

The next morning, Alyssa was less optimistic as she sat in the waiting room to see her primary care physician. She seemed to be here way too often. This was the fourth time in about six months that she had come in for one problem or another. Does your body's warranty run out at twenty? Her mom always joked that it was at age forty that everything started to fall apart. If so, Alyssa was two full decades early.

It had all started last October, when she caught strep throat after a Halloween party. It was a "famous couples" costume party, and she and her boyfriend, Caleb, had gone as Superman and Lois Lane. Unfortunately, later that night, she had seen her Superman making serious moves on a Juliet. Where was Romeo when you needed him? Alyssa and Caleb had broken up the next day, and on top of being depressed, Alyssa had developed a fever, chills, and a horrible sore throat.

She had seen Dr. Messer the next day, and after a quick swab of her throat, the doctor had told her she had strep. Alyssa had agreed to get a shot of antibiotics, rather than pills, because it was so painful to swallow. The sore throat disappeared pretty quickly, but then around a week later, she noticed a discharge on her underwear, and sometimes it burned when she urinated. Alyssa had wondered if it were possible for strep throat to somehow cause a problem "down there," but that time she didn't see the doctor. She called in and spoke with the nurse, who gave her the option of taking over-the-counter medicine to treat her symptoms. The nurse had explained that women always have both yeast and bacteria in their vaginas, and when you take an antibiotic for strep, it kills off bacteria in all parts of your body, not only in your throat. With the vaginal bacteria killed off, the yeast can overgrow, and you get a discharge. This explanation made sense, and anyway Alyssa was not anxious to have another pelvic exam besides her yearly checkup. Her symptoms improved with the over-the-counter yeast treatment, but roughly a month later, she again started having irritation and burning when she went to the bathroom.

That time, Alyssa did go to see the doctor. It was right after Thanksgiving break. She had been home in Omaha, wearing several layers of clothes to keep warm, and peeing all the time. She didn't want to say anything to her mom about her symptoms, partly because their family doctor in Nebraska was a man, and Alyssa would rather die than see a male doctor for any problem that might require a pelvic exam. Of course, Alyssa also was afraid that if she told the doctor that she'd had sex, her mother might find out. Instead, she dealt with her symptoms and hid her discomfort for a few more days. She couldn't wait to get on the plane and return to college.

Back at school, when she went to see the doctor, they skipped the pelvic anyway. Since she was complaining of urinary symptoms, the first thing the medical assistant did was to collect a urine sample. They "dipped" the urine (which means they dipped a test strip of paper into the urine to check for sugar, white blood cells, and pH levels) and then looked at it under the microscope. Apparently, Alyssa's urine had "loads" of white blood cells in it, and they treated her for a urinary tract infection without doing a pelvic exam. She took a course of antibiotics, which were the most enormous pills Alyssa had ever seen. The drugs didn't really make all of her symptoms go away, but with the busy activities of the holidays, Alyssa ignored the discomfort and went about her life.

Close to Valentine's Day, Alyssa's symptoms were being bothersome again. By then, she had tried all the home remedies for bladder infections. She was drinking tons of cranberry juice and water, so much that she had to pee constantly, even during the night. There was no way she could get any decent studying done between the lack of sleep and the numerous interruptions during the day for bathroom breaks. Alyssa went back to the doctor's office.

Again she gave a urine sample, and again it contained white blood cells. Dr. Messer asked about any vaginal symptoms and whether or not she was sexually active. Alyssa laughed and said she had sworn off guys since breaking up with Superman last year, and no, she didn't have any vaginal discharge. In truth, she *had* noticed a vaginal discharge off and on over the previous several months, but that week it seemed to be gone. "Since you had a urinary tract infection fairly recently, I'm going to give you a stronger antibiotic this time, plus we're going to culture your urine to identify specifically which bacteria you are infected with," said Dr. Messer. At least the new antibiotic was a smaller tablet than the medicine she'd taken last time. Unfortunately, three days later the nurse called Alyssa with some unexpected news.

"Hi, Alyssa, how are you feeling?," asked the nurse.

"Well, a little better, I guess," answered Alyssa.

"I'm glad you're feeling better, but we got your urine culture back, and it actually was negative," said the nurse.

"Negative? What does that mean?," asked Alyssa.

"It means you didn't have a bacterial urinary tract infection, so you can stop taking the antibiotic we prescribed. Drink plenty of water, and if your symptoms don't go away completely, then please schedule an appointment and come back in and see us, okay?"

"All right, although I can't possibly drink anymore than I've been doing already. What else could it be?," asked Alyssa.

"Maybe we need another urine culture, or perhaps you have a vaginal infection," suggested the nurse. "Be sure to follow up with us if you don't get better."

So, around ten days later, Alyssa had decided she'd better go back and get things checked out. Now that she thought about it, she had really had some irritation off and on for five or six months. She thought that maybe it had something to do with her menstrual cycle, because it seemed to get worse after each period. "Hopefully, this time, we can figure it out," she thought.

The medical assistant handed her a gown and a sheet and asked her to get changed so the doctor could examine her. Alyssa shed her clothes, put on the gown, and climbed onto the examining table. She was happy that it wasn't too cold today. While she waited, Alyssa played games on her cell phone. She was congratulating herself on finally beating a challenging level when Dr. Messer walked in.

"Hi. I'm sorry you're still having problems. Let's see if we can figure out what's going on with you, okay?," the doctor said. "What symptoms are you having?"

"Well, it's nothing awful, but I keep having irritation when I pee. It comes on for a few days, then goes away for a week or so, then comes back. Sometimes it's worse than others, but I don't understand why the antibiotics aren't working, and why the nurse told me it doesn't look like I have a bladder infection," replied Alyssa.

"Well, that's what we need to figure out," said the doctor. "Let me ask you a few more questions before I take a look at you. Have you had any fever?"

"No."

"Any back pain?"

"No."

"Nausea or vomiting?"

"Nope."

"Have you had any vaginal discharge or discomfort?," Dr. Messer asked.

Alyssa paused for a moment. "You know, I have had some off and on, but I'm not sure if the discharge has happened when I've had the burning when I pee, if that matters."

"When was the last time you had sex?"

"Gosh, a long time ago—basically Halloween," Alyssa replied. "That's too long ago to do anything, isn't it?"

"Not necessarily. Did you use condoms?," the doctor asked.

"Well, not always," Alyssa admitted.

"Sometimes sexually transmitted infections can cause urinary symptoms. Let's do a pelvic exam on you, and we'll check," said Dr. Messer. "If that is what's going on, it would certainly explain why the antibiotics didn't cure your bladder infections."

"Okay, I guess," said Alyssa, lying back and then sliding down the table. Mercifully, Dr. Messer was speedy, and the exam passed without much discomfort.

"All right. I took a sample of your discharge during the exam, and I'm going to go and look at it under the microscope while you get dressed. I'll be right back," said Dr. Messer as she stepped out of the room.

Alyssa got dressed and sat in the chair next to the table. She was about to get out her economics notes to study when there was a quick knock on the door, and Dr. Messer came back into the room.

"Well, we've got your answer, and we should definitely be able to clear up all your symptoms," the doctor said with a smile.

"What is it?," Alyssa asked.

"You've got something called trichomoniasis, or 'trich' [pronounced 'trick'] for short. It is a sexually transmitted infection, and either the second or third most common one in the United States, depending on whose statistics you use. It can take anywhere from one week to six months to show up, and it is often completely asymptomatic, so it's likely that this is the cause of your intermittent symptoms for the last several months. The previous antibiotics you took can't kill it but often will suppress the symptoms for a while. Trich is a little single-celled protozoan that is about the size of a white blood cell."

She pulled a handout from the rack on the wall and pointed to a picture of the protozoan. It looked like a fat triangle with a curly tail to Alyssa. Dr. Messer continued, "This parasite can be simple to see under the microscope if you look immediately after you take the sample, when they are still swimming. Unfortunately, if the slide sits for several minutes and dries out, it's much more difficult to pick them out if there are only a few mixed in with a bunch of white blood cells, because they're the same size and shape as those white cells. Today, as soon as I put your slide on the microscope, I saw three or four of them spinning around. Studies have shown that trich is only identified about half the time by using a microscope. It can also be identified by a culture, but not the type of standard culture that we use for urine, which is why we missed it before."

"Oh," said Alyssa, still a bit confused.

"One concern we have with trich is that it is often associated with other STIs. Some studies have shown that trich makes it easier to get other STIs, particularly HIV."

"What?!," exclaimed Alyssa. "I go from having a bladder infection to having HIV?"

"No, no, I'm not saying that you have HIV. But I am saying that having trich can increase the chance of acquiring HIV. With any STIs, including trich, we suggest testing for all STIs. I already did a swab for chlamydia and gonorrhea when I did your exam, and now we can draw your blood to test for HIV, syphilis, and hepatitis C. We'll hope that you only have trichomoniasis, but it's important to be sure."

"Okay, okay, that seems reasonable. Sorry I panicked there for a minute, but honestly, I wasn't expecting this to be an STI when I thought it was all about my bladder. Plus, I've only had sex with one guy in my whole life, and we broke up last October. It's not fair," said Alyssa, her eyes filling with tears.

"I'm sorry," said Dr. Messer. "STIs are certainly never 'fair.' The fact that you've only been with one guy definitely decreases your risk of having other STIs."

"Well, clearly Caleb gave me this, so who's to say he didn't give me something else?," Alyssa asked.

"Unfortunately, you are correct about that, which is why we're going to test you for everything, to be sure. Anyway, the good news is that we definitely can cure trich. Here is a prescription for an antibiotic called metronidazole. You take one pill twice per day for a week. There is a single-dose method too, but I find that it tends to cause more side effects. Make sure you don't drink any alcohol at all while you are on this medicine, because that can cause a miserable reaction with severe nausea and vomiting. Of course, your ex will likely need to be treated too, so he doesn't spread this to anyone else."

"Um... how does that work? Do I give you his name, and someone calls him?," Alyssa asked hopefully.

"No, I'm sorry. I'm afraid you have the pleasure of making that phone call. Many people prefer to send an email or text. If you want to send him information, there's a link to an excellent website on the pamphlet," said Dr. Messer.

"Wouldn't he know that he has this? What happens in guys?," asked Alyssa.

"Unfortunately, this disease gets spread easily partly because there are no symptoms, especially in men. So it's entirely possible that Caleb has no clue that he has trich or that he gave it to you," answered Dr. Messer.

"Can't you give me a prescription to give to him?," asked Alyssa, thinking to herself that there was no way Caleb would actually go to a doctor. She didn't care much about him at this point, but she did feel sorry for anyone else he had slept with. Well, maybe not for "Juliet," but for others.

"No, I cannot legally do that in this state. We have to leave it up to you to tell him, and he has to go to a doctor to get treatment. Sorry. Do you have any other questions?," Dr. Messer asked.

"When will I have the results of the other tests?"

"Usually they're ready in about three days. We will notify you via email that you have a secure message with your results, so you can log in to our system and see them."

"Do I need a follow-up appointment?," asked Alyssa.

"Probably not. Assuming your other tests are all negative, this antibiotic should fix your symptoms for good. Of course, if you have any other concerns, please come back," said the doctor with a smile.

Alyssa stood and gathered her things. With her usual sense of humor beginning to sneak back in, she turned to Dr. Messer and grinned. "You know, the last time I went out with Caleb was Halloween. I guess you're 'treating' my 'trich.'"

They shared a chuckle, both thinking that next Halloween the phrase "trick or treat" would have a different meaning.

12: Sean

SEAN SQUINTED AT HIS phone and saw the time: 9:52. "No way!," he panicked, simultaneously leaping out of bed and pulling on his jeans. "I can still make it to my test on time if I run," he rationalized. After staying awake to study past 3 a.m., he had apparently slept through his alarm. Sean grabbed his backpack and flew out of the dorm. Luckily, the chemistry building was close enough that Sean made it there only a few minutes late, sliding into his seat in time to hear the final instructions for the test.

"And please, everyone, double-check that your cell phones are silenced," announced the professor.

Dutifully, Sean fished in his backpack for his phone and, glancing at the screen, was startled to see a text from his former girlfriend. "We need to talk asap."

"What, no emojis?," was Sean's immediate reaction, briefly smiling at the memory of his fiery, redheaded ex and her boundless enthusiasm.

As a high school couple, Sean and Jen were awesome. However, they had followed scholarship opportunities that landed them at separate universities, and the long-distance relationship challenges were overwhelming. Jen broke up with Sean during Christmas break when she found out Sean had not stayed faithful. Sean felt badly that his cheating caused the end of their relationship; however, he maintained that college was the right time to meet other people and casually date around before making a serious commitment. Of course, his definition of "casually dating around" had proven to be quite different than Jen's.

Sean's mind jumped back to the present as he broke the seal to open his test booklet, and thoughts of Jen vanished as he focused on equations and chemical properties.

After the test, Sean grabbed a soda and texted Jen: "What's up?"

Sean had barely sent the text when he felt his phone vibrating with an incoming call. "Sean, I'm going to kill you," Jen whispered fiercely. "Hold on a second while I get to where I can talk."

"And a cheery good morning to you too, Jen," Sean countered. "Don't get all pissed at me. You're the one who wanted to talk."

"I am furious at you," hissed Jen. "Hold on a second."

"The nerve of her," Sean thought, irritated to the core. Out loud, he said, "What can I possibly have done to upset you now? We haven't even seen or talked to each other in four months."

"Okay, I'm outside. Now I can talk. Look, I appreciate you texting back. I know I shouldn't have started the phone call like that, but Sean, I am so pissed at you," Jen responded.

"You've clearly established that, but perhaps you'd like to share why you're so upset?," said Sean in an overly polite tone.

"Yes, I'd love to share, as apparently you did," said Jen, mimicking his tone.

"What are you trying to tell me, Jen?," asked Sean.

"You gave me a disease, a sexually transmitted infection, to be exact!," accused Jen.

"Yeah, right," snorted Sean.

"Sean, I'm serious. I've been having lots of problems off and on since Christmas, and this morning I found out that it's all from trichomoniasis," explained Jen.

"Trich-a-what?," asked Sean, still confused.

"Trichomoniasis, Mr. Pre-Med," said Jen angrily. "Put in your language, trich is a single-celled parasite that apparently is the most common nonviral sexually transmitted infection."

"Listen, Jen, I don't know who else you've been with, but I most certainly do not have any infection," retorted Sean.

"I have not 'been with' anyone except you, dear Sean. So, unlike you, I don't need to rack my brain to figure out where this came from," spat Jen.

Sean knew enough about Jen to believe that her statement was true. They were both virgins when they decided to have sex back in high school, and he was definitely the one who had pushed that issue. Sean would have been surprised and disappointed if Jen had already slept with someone else. Still, the whole idea of him giving her an STI seemed farfetched. He'd only been with a couple of other girls. "But I don't have any symptoms of anything," he protested.

"My doctor told me that ninety percent of men have no symptoms, so that's not surprising. Not all women get symptoms, but I guess I was *lucky*," said Jen.

"Did they give you something to treat it?," asked Sean.

"Yes, so I guess now I'm actually fixed, but I thought you might want to know that you have this infection," said Jen bitterly.

"Well, I'm sorry, but I'm not convinced that I do have it," said Sean.

"Let me make this as clear as possible. There is *no other way I could have caught trich*, except from you. You are the one and only guy who has been anywhere near me when I was not wearing clothes. I have certainly kissed a few other guys, Sean, but nothing else. Not from their lack of trying, I might add," she finished.

"I know, I know. But seriously, you can't expect me to feel guilty about something I never even knew that I had," said Sean defensively.

"Frankly, I don't expect anything from you anymore," retorted Jen. "Let's not prolong this conversation. I'm trying to do the right thing by telling you about the trich. I don't want any other girls to get this disease, regardless of what I may think of your new companions. Please promise me that you will go to the doctor and get treated. I think you owe me that, Sean."

"Jen, it's not like I'm sleeping around a ton."

"Honestly, I don't even want to know. Let's not do this to each other. Go to the doctor and get the antibiotics. They're not too much fun to take, but you'll be cured. I've got to get back to class. Goodbye, Sean," she said definitively.

"Bye, and I'm sorry," Sean replied. This day was not going well.

A few days later, Sean was sitting in the health center, waiting to see a doctor. After reading everything about trich on what he thought were reliable websites, like the Centers for Disease Control and the National Institutes of Health, Sean was convinced that he ought to get treated. He actually still hoped to see Jen this summer when they were both home from school, and he knew he wouldn't be able to look her in the eye unless he'd received treatment.

"Sean?," called out a cute medical assistant holding a clipboard.

Sean stood up. "That's me," he said, gathering his backpack and following her down the hall.

The aide chatted as she weighed Sean and took his blood pressure and pulse. "Hi, Sean, I'm Nicole. I'm a medical assistant here at the clinic. Aren't you in the pre-med club? I think I recognize you from the last meeting."

"Oh, great," thought Sean, "this is so not the moment I want to be recognized." He did think that Nicole's face looked familiar, with her hazel eyes and light brown hair pulled back into a ponytail. Nicole's dark blue scrubs, the uniform of the clinic, took away any other sense of recognition. "I was at the last meeting, but I haven't decided about joining. Everyone seemed pretty intense," said Sean, trying to shift the focus away from himself.

"Oh, that's because the juniors and seniors were all hyped about the MCAT. I think that meeting was right before the last test, and you know if you bomb that admissions test you can kiss your dreams of med school goodbye," Nicole explained. "You really should give it another try before you decide." Nicole finished writing down Sean's vital signs and then asked, "So, what brings you in today?"

Sean stammered, "I... I wanted to talk to the doctor about getting a prescription filled, that's all. Thanks for getting me all checked in," he smiled convincingly.

"Okay, sure. What prescription?," Nicole inquired.

"Um, it's an antibiotic for skin stuff," Sean lied, hoping she would believe him. On the appointment request, he had simply checked "medication issue" because he was embarrassed to put "STI screening."

"Do you remember the name?," she asked.

"Sorry, no I don't. I thought I could talk to the doctor about different treatment options," Sean murmured.

Luckily, Nicole had worked at the clinic long enough to know not to press any further. Sean sat in the chair and searched on his phone for WebMD so he could review the trichomoniasis information. He figured that as a pre-med student, it would be good to at least seem informed. The doctor entered before Sean made it all the way through the webpage.

"Hello, Sean, I'm Dr. Kwun," the doctor introduced herself and then sat on her stool and logged in to the computer. Dr. Kwun was wearing a dark suit under her starched white lab coat. She spoke softly and deliberately. "Looks like you've got some questions for me about a medication refill?"

"Well, not exactly. I do need an antibiotic, but not for acne. To be honest, it's for something kind of embarrassing."

Dr. Kwun nodded, indicating she was listening.

"My ex-girlfriend has been diagnosed with trichomoniasis, and well, I'm the only person that, um, that..."

"That she's been intimate with?," Dr. Kwun finished.

"Exactly," said Sean.

"But I'm assuming that you have had other partners," added Dr. Kwun dryly.

"Right," confirmed Sean.

"And what have you been using for protection?," asked Dr. Kwun.

"Jen, my old girlfriend, was on the pill, so we didn't use anything else. I've only been with a couple of other girls, and I used condoms," said Sean.

"Consistently?," asked Dr. Kwun.

Sean couldn't read Dr. Kwun at all. Her even tone and neutral expression hid any indication of what she was thinking. "Apparently not," Sean admitted. He wanted to add that he was not the type of guy who mindlessly sleeps with any girl available, but he felt the need to match Dr. Kwun's somewhat detached manner.

"I see you are a pre-med major, is that correct?," inquired Dr. Kwun.

"Yes," nodded Sean.

"I hate to make assumptions, but with your major, I'm guessing you might have done some Internet research about trichomoniasis. Is that correct?"

Sean nodded again, adding, "I tried to stick to reliable sites like WebMD and the CDC."

"Good for you. There is a ton of misinformation on the web, but those are indeed reputable sites that should have provided you with solid basic information about trich. As I am sure you are now aware, trichomoniasis is a parasite that is only transmitted through direct genital-to-genital contact. Since your ex presumably contracted trich from you, we need to move forward with treatment and further testing," said Dr. Kwun.

"Further testing?," asked Sean. "Actually, my impression from reading this stuff was that since the testing is not very reliable in men, you would automatically treat me."

"For trich, yes, you're absolutely right. Men only test positive around half of the time that they actually have the infection, so we treat all sexual partners of anyone confirmed with trich. I was referring to additional testing to make sure you don't have other sexually transmitted infections as well."

"But I don't have any symptoms at all," said Sean, petulant and now anxious, since he hadn't yet made that leap of logic.

"The majority of STIs are asymptomatic in men, as I imagine you found in your research," replied Dr. Kwun. "Today, I will perform a brief physical exam, and then we can draw your blood to test for HIV and syphilis, plus check your urine for chlamydia and gonorrhea. We can also test for trichomoniasis if you would like, but as you read online, treatment is recommended even in the presence of a negative test if your partner has a confirmed case."

"If it's not too expensive, I would like you to go ahead and test me, if only for academic curiosity," said Sean.

"My assistant can check the cost of the test and let you know, so you can make a decision," agreed Dr. Kwun. "Let me step outside while you get undressed from the waist down, and sit up here with this drape over your legs. Nicole and I will be back to complete your STI testing in a moment."

"Dr. Kwun, does Nicole have to assist you?," asked Sean quickly. "I kind of know her, and it would be really awkward for me."

"I understand. If there is another medical assistant available, I will bring them instead," she responded. "Per our clinic's policy, we must have a chaperone in the room for any genital exam on men or breast or pelvic exams on women. Please get changed."

Sean quickly shed his jeans and underwear, following her directions with the drape. "How humiliated can I get?," he wondered, feeling quite vulnerable, naked beneath the sheet. Before long, Dr. Kwun returned, followed by a tall, wiry young man wearing dark blue scrubs like the ones Nicole had on.

"This is Michael. He'll be assisting me," said Dr. Kwun, her voice unchanged.

"Thanks," mumbled Sean.

Michael seemed a bit flustered as he pulled out an assortment of tubes and swabs, and set them on the side table tray. Dr. Kwun seemed to take no notice of Michael and simply indicated that Sean should lie back as she slid out a hidden portion at the end of the exam table, extending the length to accommodate Sean's legs and feet. She lifted the drape and deftly examined Sean's abdomen, pubic area, penis, and testicles.

"Everything appears normal today on your exam. There are no obvious signs of pubic lice, genital warts, or herpes. Your testicles feel normal as well—no bumps that might indicate a concern for testicular cancer. You may or may not already know that testicular cancer occurs most commonly in men in their twenties. It may show up as a painless lump or swelling in one testicle, so come in for an exam immediately if that ever occurs," instructed Dr. Kwun.

Sean nodded and then, glancing at the side table, inquired, "Do you have to get a . . . sample of anything to test me?"

The doctor shook her head. "No. We use those swabs if there is an ulcer suggestive of herpes, or to assess any obvious penile discharge, but you have neither. After you get dressed we will send you over to the lab to have your blood drawn and give a urine sample," stated Dr. Kwun.

"Are you going to check my blood for herpes too?," asked Sean.

"Herpes is not part of our standard panel, but we can certainly add that to your lab orders if you would like," she replied.

"Why not?"

"There are multiple factors, but the main reasons are that the test is relatively expensive, it's a silent disease that is extremely common, and there is debate in the medical literature about the role of herpes antibody testing. The CDC, for example, does not recommend herpes blood tests for general screening, but does recommend type-specific herpes blood testing for patients presenting for an evaluation of a sexually transmitted infection, such as yourself. Would you like me to add it?," she asked.

"Uh, yes, please. I might as well check everything. Are we done here?," asked Sean hopefully, leaning forward to sit up.

"Yes, except for giving you a prescription to treat your trich," she replied, sliding the leg extender back into the table and motioning for Sean to sit up as she moved back over to the computer. "I should have asked this earlier, but did your ex-girlfriend or any of your other sexual partners test positive for anything else?"

"No," he responded, blushing. At the thought of Jen, Sean was flooded with guilt. Poor Jen, she hadn't done anything to deserve this. He imagined her embarrassment and fury after going through this routine only to be told that she had an STI. She must really hate him.

"Do you tolerate medicine well?," asked Dr. Kwun as she pulled out her prescription pad.

"What do you mean?," asked Sean, confused. "I don't often take medicines."

"This particular medicine can cause a metallic taste in your mouth, nausea, abdominal cramping, and/or headaches. We have a choice of giving you a single large dose or seven days of a smaller dose. The single dose has more side effects, but obviously ends more quickly. Also, you can't have any alcohol during treatment, or for three days afterward," Dr. Kwun rattled off.

"Three days?," said Sean, thinking about the upcoming weekend.

"Yes, because when this antibiotic combines with alcohol in your system, it can cause severe abdominal cramps, nausea, vomiting, headaches, and flushing. That's why the drug company recommends avoiding alcohol for three days after you finish your last dose, in order to be sure the medication is out of your system. Volunteer to be the designated driver for a week," suggested Dr. Kwun.

"Not to be a pain," Sean said, "but I read that the extended-release form of the medicine doesn't cause as many side effects. Can I get that?"

"Not from our pharmacy. We only stock the generic," Dr. Kwun replied evenly. "But I can print out a prescription if you would like to take it to another pharmacy. Which treatment would you prefer: single dose, week-long dose of generic twice daily, or week-long once daily extended release?"

Sean paused. He was beginning to understand Jen's words when she said the treatment wasn't "too much fun to take." Sean actually had a very sensitive stomach, at least when it came to new foods or stress. He didn't remember ever taking a medicine that made him feel badly, but then again, he couldn't remember the last time he was even sick. Choosing between a week of possible low-grade symptoms and a couple of days of potentially feeling really crappy was not a great choice. Add in no beer for ten days, with his birthday coming next week, and the decision only got worse.

"Well?," Dr. Kwun asked.

"I guess I'll take the single dose," answered Sean. "Are they all equally effective?"

"No, they're not. We use the seven-day treatment if the single dose fails. However, in our clinic, the single dose works the vast majority of the time," said Dr. Kwun. "Most of the recurrences we see appear to be from partners not getting treated."

"I certainly don't want to take it more than once," Sean mused, "but I don't want to be sick for a week either." He couldn't decide.

"Do you want to use our pharmacy?," she asked, fingers poised over the keyboard.

"Yes, please."

"How about if I write the prescription so you can decide later? The pharmacist will give you fourteen pills. Take one pill twice per day for seven days. Or, if you'd prefer, you can choose to take four pills all at once. Please make certain that you complete a full course, one way or another. Throw away the extra tablets if you take the single dose. *Do not give them away, as they can have very dangerous interactions.*" She typed in the prescription. "I sent it electronically to our pharmacy. You may check out at the front desk, then head over to the lab. You will be notified when your results are available in approximately three or four days. Please send in your other partners to be treated as well. Any questions?"

Sean shook his head. "No, I think that covers it. Thanks."

Dr. Kwun and Michael left the room, leaving Sean to get dressed.

"Send in your other partners," Dr. Kwun had said, reminding Sean that he had been focused so much on Jen that he hadn't even thought about who gave trich to him in the first place. Sean had slept with two different young women besides Jen last semester, neither of whom he had spoken to in over six months.

Sean had no desire to contact either woman. The first, Peyton, didn't even attend school here. Sean thought she was a relative or friend of his roommate's girlfriend. Peyton had showed up to a dorm party the second week of school. She was older, experienced, willing, and able. But looking back, Sean couldn't imagine why he had sex with her. "I must have been so surprised to have an open invitation that I acted without thinking. I'd lay money down that she's the source of this trich," he thought, mentally kicking himself.

Brooke, the second girl, had been more of a buddy to him. While celebrating after a football game one night, Brooke threw herself at Sean, pouring out her feelings and trying to convince him she could be a better match than Jen. That hookup lasted about a week, until Sean decided he still had deep feelings for Jen. Unfortunately, Brooke had hung on and repeatedly called him in tears, begging him to give her another chance. Sean thought any communication with Brooke could be disastrous. "Then again," Sean thought, "telling Brooke I likely gave her an STI certainly shouldn't stir up any flames of desire from her."

Sean finished tying his shoes and slung his backpack over his shoulder. The blood draw at the lab went smoothly, but the pharmacy was packed. He chose not to hang around until the prescription was ready but planned to come back the next day to pick it up. He was still undecided about which treatment to take. "I wonder which one Jen took," Sean thought. He truly felt awful about giving her an STI and wanted to somehow make it up to her. Sean knew she was too angry with him to talk, but he had to do something. Should he send her flowers? Or maybe Jen's favorite, Tiff's Treats chocolate chip cookies? How do you tell someone you are truly, truly sorry for something like this? No treat in the world would be enough... but he would start with flowers, in case Jen's stomach was still messed up from the antibiotics.

facts

Trichomoniasis Fact Sheet

What is it?

- Trichomoniasis ("trich" for short) is caused by a single-celled protozoan parasite called Trichomonas vaginalis.

How common is it?

- CDC estimates suggest that 3.7 million people are infected in the United States each year.

- Trichomoniasis is thought to be the most common nonviral STI, but significant racial disparity exists: non-Hispanic white women: 1.8%; Mexican American women: 1.3%; non-Hispanic black women: 13.3%.

How do you get it?

- Trich is transmitted by direct genital-to-genital contact, including but not limited to intercourse.

Where on your body do you get it?

- Trich infects the urogenital tract.
- In women, the vagina is the most common location.
- In men, the urethra is the most common site.

How do I know if I have it?

- Many people are asymptomatic.
- Diagnosis is often difficult, because current tests have low sensitivities, ranging from 24% to 83%. This means that nearly half the time the infection is present, the tests fail to show a positive result.
- Pap smears may coincidentally identify trich (but only with 24% sensitivity, meaning that it is detected only 24% of the time that it is actually present).

What does it look like?

- Normal anatomy.
- Yellow-green or gray discharge in the vagina.
- Redness or small sores on the cervix (seen by the physician during an exam with a speculum).

What does it feel like?

- Most men and many women are unaware they have trich.
- 90% of men have no symptoms. In the 10% of men with symptoms, most complain of urethral discharge and/or pain with urination or ejaculation.
- Women may have dyspareunia (painful intercourse).
- Women may notice a bad odor, itching, and/or yellow-green or gray heavy, frothy discharge from the vagina.

How long does it last?

- Trich lasts until it is treated with appropriate antibiotics.
- If symptomatic, it usually manifests between 5 and 28 days from initial contact, but symptoms may come and go, making it difficult to identify a time frame.

Can it be cured?

- Yes, although there is increasing resistance to metronidazole.

Can you be reinfected?

- Yes, you can be reinfected.
- Reinfection is common when a partner is not fully treated.

What is the treatment?

- The drug of choice is metronidazole (Flagyl), which can be given as a single 2 g dose or as a 500 mg tablet taken twice per day for one week.

- Metronidazole has a high incidence of side effects, including nausea, vomiting, headaches, loss of appetite, and metallic taste.
- A person taking metronidazole must abstain from alcohol in all forms during treatment and for three days afterward.
- The only other drug indicated for trich is tinidazole (Tindamax and Fasigyn), given as a 2 g single dose; no alcohol should be consumed for three days after completion of treatment with this drug.
- If a single-dose treatment fails to eliminate symptoms, and reinfection is excluded, then seven days of therapy with metronidazole, 500 mg twice per day, is recommended.
- All sex partners should be treated.

How about alternative therapies?

- Douching is definitely not helpful and likely harmful.
- No herbs or other nonprescription remedies have been proven to eliminate trich.

Are there long-term consequences?

- Trich is associated with giving birth to premature and low-birth-weight infants.
- Trich has been linked with a threefold to fivefold increase in the transmission or acquisition of HIV.
- Trich is linked with increased risk of infertility and PID (pelvic inflammatory disease).

When are you contagious?

- If you are infected, you are contagious until you are fully treated.
- Latex male condoms can reduce but not eliminate transmission of trich.

How do I avoid getting trich?

- Abstaining from intercourse and from direct genital-to-genital contact will prevent the transmission of trich.
- Using male condoms will decrease but not eliminate the transmission of trich.
- Use new condoms on shared sex toys for each partner or, preferably, do not share sex toys.

If I have trich, how do I avoid giving it to my partner?

- If you have had no prior sexual contact with your partner, abstain from sex and direct genital-to-genital contact until you have completed appropriate antibiotic therapy.
- If you have had prior sexual intimacy with your partner, abstain from sex and from direct genital-to-genital contact until you both have completed antibiotic treatment for trich.

Can trich be passed through homosexual contact?

- Since it is not transmitted through oral or anal sex, male-to-male transmission is very unlikely.
- There is evidence of vulva-to-vulva transmission as well as transmission through shared sex toys in women.

Frequently Asked Questions

➤ **Did I catch trich from a toilet seat?**
No. Although the parasite has been found on damp towels and underwear, transmission other than by direct genital contact has never been documented.

➤ **Did I get trich from oral or anal sex?**
No. Trich cannot survive in the mouth or anus.

➤ **If I just developed symptoms, is it from my current partner?**
Possibly. Women who develop symptoms most often begin to have complaints in 4–28 days after exposure, or they may remain asymptomatic for a long period of time.

➤ **If I caught it from my current partner, is he cheating on me?**
Not necessarily. Since men are almost always asymptomatic, they may have been infected for a long time without knowing it.

Additional Information

American College of Obstetricians and Gynecologists
PO Box 70620
Washington, DC 20024-9998
1-800-673-8444
www.acog.org/publications/patient_education/bp009.cfm

American Sexual Health Association
PO Box 13827
Research Triangle Park, NC 27709
919-361-8400
www.ashasexualhealth.org/

Centers for Disease Control and Prevention
1600 Clifton Road
Atlanta, GA 30329-4027

1-800-CDC-INFO (1-800-232-4636), 1-888-232-6348 (TTY)
www.cdc.gov/ncidod/dpd/parasites/trichomoniasis.htm

MedlinePlus
US National Library of Medicine
8600 Rockville Pike
Bethesda, MD 20894
1-888-FIND-NLM (1-888-346-3656) or 301-594-5983
www.nlm.nih.gov/medlineplus/trichomoniasis.html

PUBIC LICE

13: Zoe

ZOE RELAXED INTO THE rhythm of massaging her client's thick blonde hair with the rich lather of her favorite shampoo. "You've picked up quite a few natural highlights," she commented.

"You wouldn't believe how hot it was down in Cancun last week," lamented Jason. "I would have melted if the frozen drinks didn't cool me down."

"And this was supposedly work?," said Zoe. "I could have sworn you said you were going to Mexico for business."

"Well, entertaining clients is business," Jason defended himself. "That's what the world of sales is all about."

"Tough life," joked Zoe, as she rinsed his hair.

"Yeah, but someone's got to do it," Jason replied.

Zoe finished towel-drying his hair. "Okay, follow me to my station."

Jason followed, checking out her tight-fitting pants along the way, and sat down in the leather chair. "Hey look, you match the chair," Jason teased. "Both black leather."

"Yeah, but I sit in cute guys' laps, not the other way around," rebutted Zoe.

This was the fourth time Zoe had cut Jason's hair, and the chemistry between them was simmering. As she leaned forward and brushed off the loose hairs on the cape covering his torso, Zoe was busily trying to think of a subtle way to let him know she was available.

"Hey, Zoe, who are you taking to the after-party tonight?," asked her co-worker Linda as she walked past Zoe's station.

It was exactly the opening she needed. "Oh, you know me, I'd rather fly solo," Zoe said breezily, gratefully answering in Linda's direction but secretly looking in the mirror for any response from Jason.

"So you don't have a boyfriend right now?," interjected Jason.

Zoe laughed casually. "Nope, too much work. I'm committed to no one. How about you?"

Jason smiled. "I travel too much to get tied down." They continued their banter through his haircut. When he was ready to leave, Jason handed Zoe his business card. "The bottom number is my cell phone. Why don't you text me if you want company at that after-party your friend mentioned?"

"Seriously?," Zoe asked, suddenly nervous.

"Absolutely," reassured Jason. "I have a late meeting 'til roughly eight, but then I'm free. Text me and let me know where to meet you."

"Sounds great," Zoe confirmed happily.

After Jason left, the afternoon passed quickly. Linda and Francisco walked over as Zoe was cleaning up her station. "Ah, Jason, the man with the golden hair," teased Linda. "Kind of like that Jason from mythology with the golden fleece, right?"

"Are you comparing him with a sheep?," laughed Zoe. "I'd like to think his mane is far superior to the hair of a barnyard animal."

"And hopefully much cleaner," added Francisco, brushing back his purple-streaked hair.

"And less fragrant," finished Linda, holding her nose.

"This conversation has degenerated," announced Zoe. "Come on, Linda, if you're riding with me, let's go."

Before long, Linda and Zoe had transformed themselves. They were now wearing their favorite party outfits complete with flawless makeup and perfectly styled hair, and were driving over to meet the rest of their friends at Club 21. Earlier, Zoe had texted Jason where and when to meet up, and she was pleased to see him already at the bar, standing next to Francisco and a few of her other co-workers.

"Hey! Glad you recognized my friends," said Zoe as she walked up.

"Francisco definitely stands out in a crowd," commented Jason, referring to Francisco's flamboyant style.

"And, of course, we spotted Golden Boy and called him right over," said Francisco, stroking Jason's arm.

"No stealing my date," Zoe scolded, stepping between the two of them and slipping her arm around Jason's waist.

"You know I'd love to, but trust me, I'm not his type," Francisco responded with a lewd glance at Jason.

Jason looked very uncomfortable. "Yeah, I prefer . . . blondes," he said with a weak smile. "Seriously, I'm glad you're here, Zoe. I'm usually up for the club scene, but after being stuck in meetings all day, this pounding music and the flashing lights are a bit overstimulating. How about you and I sneak out to my place instead? I have a fully stocked bar, and we can order takeout from anywhere you'd like."

"Sounds great to me," said Zoe. "Let's go."

"No fair, already heading to Golden Boy's stable," whined Linda discreetly as Zoe handed over the car keys. "See you tomorrow."

"Gee, was it something I said?," Francisco joked.

The next day Zoe was grilled at work.

"How was your date?," asked Amy, the colorist.

"I'll bet he was as yummy as he looks," offered Francisco.

"More importantly, does he have any friends?," asked Linda.

"Really, guys, back off. Jason is cute enough, but I think he's too conservative for me," Zoe answered. "And I think he was a bit put off by our crowd."

"So did you sleep with him?," persisted Francisco, ever the gossip.

"Yes, not that it's any of your business," laughed Zoe.

"And did you use protection?," Francisco demanded, hands on his hips.

"Of course!," Zoe said with an eye roll. "I will give him credit, he supplied the condoms, though I had some in my purse. This guy is a neat freak. I swear that his apartment looks like he has hourly maid service. Even his bed was perfectly made up." She paused. "But to be honest, I'm not that into him. He's all about *Newsweek* and stock futures, and I'm more about enjoying the here and now for a few more years."

"So you aren't going to go out with him again?," asked Amy.

Zoe shook her head. "I don't think so. Not unless I need a date to a family function. He's the kind of guy they'd think was perfect for me."

Two nights later, lying in bed, the image of Jason in his bed was foremost in Zoe's mind as she found herself repeatedly scratching her pubic area. "This itch is driving me nuts," thought Zoe. "It's worse than last night." She vaguely remembered Jason scratching his crotch during the night but had written it off as a rude male habit. "Maybe I'm imagining the worst, but I've got to get this checked out. I'm going to claw myself to death."

The next morning, Zoe was able to get an early walk-in appointment with her family doctor. Dr. Patel was always full of energy and meticulously dressed. Zoe was not her stylist, but she appreciated Dr. Patel's chin-length bob, which worked well with her thick dark hair.

"Hi, Zoe," greeted Dr. Patel as she entered the exam room. "What brings you in today?"

"Hi, Dr. Patel. Nice haircut," Zoe complimented. "It's kind of embarrassing, but I'm here because I've got an unbelievably itchy crotch."

"Is there a rash?," asked the doctor.

"I didn't see one," answered Zoe.

"How long have you been itchy?"

"Just the last few days."

"Are you using new laundry detergent? Or any new soaps, gels, lotions, or shampoos?," quizzed Dr. Patel.

"I did get a new bath gel last week," mused Zoe.

"But the only spot you're itching is your groin?," verified the physician.

"Well, sometimes I'm itching all over, but I think that's in my head. The only part that is driving me nuts is my crotch," said Zoe.

"Any vaginal discharge or burning when you pee?"

"None."

"Any new sexual partners?," Dr. Patel inquired.

"Only one," admitted Zoe.

"You know that's all it takes, Zoe. Did you use protection beyond your birth control pill?"

"Of course. I always use condoms."

"Good for you. Remember, condoms can't protect against everything though, so consider getting tested for STIs today after we look at you. Ready?," said Dr. Patel. Zoe was already dressed in a patient gown, without underwear, as the nurse had instructed. She lay back for the doctor to examine her.

"I can see where you've been scratching," commented the doctor as she looked at Zoe. Dr. Patel pulled over a large magnifying glass with a built-in lamp that looked exactly like the one Zoe's mom used when she did needlepoint. "This helps my rapidly aging eyes," she joked as she continued her exam. "Oh, here's the problem. Zoe, brace yourself, because you're not going to like this. It looks like you've got pubic lice. I'm going to go look at one of your hairs under the microscope, but I believe these are nits."

Zoe recoiled. "Gross. If there is one thing hair stylists can't stand, it's lice. Oh man, I'm definitely going to itch everywhere now."

"I'll be right back," said Dr. Patel, leaving the room with the hair in her gloved hands.

Zoe sat up and looked through the magnifying lens that was still suspended over her crotch. She did not need the doctor's confirmation: indeed, her pubic hair had multiple nits. Zoe was disgusted, but she started picking at and removing the nits with her fingernails.

Dr. Patel returned to find Zoe busily extracting nits. "Sorry, Zoe, but as apparently you can see, it's definitely pubic lice nits, better known as crabs."

"Dr. Patel, our worst nightmare at the salon is one of our clients bringing in their daughter with a thick head of hair all full of lice, asking us to give them the cutest, shortest haircut possible. We call them 'pediculosis princesses.' It happens every month or two, and we all walk around scratching our heads for a week afterward," shuddered Zoe.

"I understand. At least this is a much smaller area to cover," the doctor said optimistically.

"But way more disgusting," disagreed Zoe. "Ironically, I actually washed this guy's hair before our date. He was my client. I can assure you that he didn't have any lice on his head. Isn't it the same bug?"

"No, surprisingly, it's not. Pubic lice strongly prefer the coarse pubic hair, and only branch out to axillary hair, eyelashes, or beards and mustaches."

"Axillary?," questioned Zoe.

"Armpits."

Zoe quickly crossed her arms as though to protect her armpits from invasion, a look of revulsion on her face. "Yuck. I assume I know who gave me this, but where do most people get them? This guy I went out with has excellent hygiene, and his place was unbelievably clean. I'm sure he must have a maid. He is the last person I would suspect to have lice."

"Does he travel?," asked the doctor.

"Yes, he says that he travels a ton for his job. In fact, he just got back from Mexico," said Zoe.

"Perhaps he got it from hotel linens that were infected and not adequately cleaned," said Dr. Patel.

Zoe shrugged. "All I really want to know at this point is, how do I get rid of them?"

"Well, there are several over-the-counter products to choose from," said Dr. Patel. "We generally don't use the prescription medicine, lindane, unless the other products don't work, because it has more side effects."

"I want the strongest one that works the best," pleaded Zoe. "Please go ahead and give me the prescription one. I don't want these nasty little crabs one minute longer than I absolutely have to deal with them."

"Well, you're not pregnant, nursing, or too young, and you don't have any open sores, so there shouldn't be any problem with that,"

Dr. Patel reasoned out loud as she sat at the computer and started typing. "Are you still using CVS Pharmacy on Main Street for your prescriptions?"

Zoe nodded. "Yes. Are you sending it now? I am going straight there so I can get rid of this as soon as possible."

"I am, but really, I'd recommend the over-the-counter products. If they don't work, then fill this prescription. Follow the directions exactly. More is not better in this case. You only leave the shampoo on for four minutes, then rinse it off thoroughly. Finish picking off the nits after you shampoo. The most important part is treating all your linens as well. Wash your towels, sheets, blankets, and clothes in hot soapy water, and then dry them in a dryer for at least twenty minutes. If you have anything in those categories that can't be washed and dried, bag them up in sealed plastic bags and leave them there for fourteen days," the doctor instructed.

"No way. I'm throwing everything out," said Zoe. "I've been looking for an excuse to get new bedding, and this is it."

"I wouldn't get new stuff until you're sure you are completely treated," cautioned the doctor. "Some people need a second treatment a week or so later. The medicine only kills the adult form of the lice. If any eggs are missed when you manually remove the nits, they will hatch in about a week and restart the cycle."

"How long do they live?," asked Zoe.

"Eggs—the nits—last roughly seven days, then nymphs, which are immature adults, crawl out. It takes another week for the nymphs to become adult lice capable of laying eggs. An adult female lays up to ten eggs per day and lives roughly two weeks. Adult lice can only survive one to two days off a human though."

"What about my couch and chairs?," asked Zoe.

"Assuming you've only sat on your couch in clothes, it's not a problem. If you slept on it in just underwear, I'd spray it with an over-the-counter anti-lice spray," answered the doctor.

"When will I stop itching?"

"The itch often stays for several days after you've completed treatment. Don't worry about it unless you continue to see nits. Sometimes putting calamine lotion on the itchy spots will help, or taking an oral antihistamine like diphenhydramine, which is

Benadryl, at bedtime will help calm down the itch and let you sleep easier." Dr. Patel paused. "Remember to let your friend from the other night know, so he can get treated too. And let's draw your blood and have you give us a urine sample so we can be sure he didn't share anything else with you."

"You can be sure I'll let him know. And yes, please go ahead and check me for everything."

As she got dressed, her friends' barnyard jokes popped back into her head. "Maybe he does belong on a farm," Zoe thought. She could only imagine the new nicknames Jason would have at the salon. Golden Boy would be out, replaced with Pediculosis Prince, Lice Lord, Crab Crotch, or worse. Good thing she wasn't hooked on him. Heaven help him if he ever returned for a haircut. She pulled out her cell phone and searched for his number.

"Okay, Jason," she smirked as her thumbs flew across her keyboard. "Hey, got a new hair product that you really need. Text me."

14: Ryan

"PROMISE ME THAT YOU won't do anything stupid just to impress all your buddies," Elise begged. "I know how you all try to out-macho one another, especially after a few beers."

Ryan rolled his eyes, glad that his fiancée wasn't able to see his expression as he spoke into his cell phone. "Really, everything will be fine. Don't get so worked up. It's more about a guys weekend hanging out at the lake than the bachelor party," he said.

"Look, you know I'm not the typical hysterical bride," Elise replied calmly, "but I can picture Nick or Chris getting you all to jump in the lake for a midnight swim or something after you've been drinking all night, and I don't want you to drown or break an arm."

"Don't worry. The strippers will be there before midnight, so no one will want to leave the house," Ryan joked, as the passengers in his car erupted in laughter.

"Okay, now you're pushing your luck. You know I trust you, Ryan, but your high school friends are another deal," Elise warned.

"I'm teasing, Elise. Go enjoy your girls spa weekend and relax with all the pampering your heart desires. I promise to keep the guys under control, or if I can't do that, I at least promise to lock myself in a room away from them." Ryan laughed.

"Fair enough," sighed Elise. "Have fun and be safe. I love you."

"Love you too," responded Ryan in a whisper, and he quickly hung up.

A falsetto chorus of "We love you too" echoed throughout the car from Ryan's groomsmen. Who knew what this weekend would bring?

The caravan pulled up to Nick's lake house, and young men poured out of several cars. "Ah, the famous love shack of the not-so-famous Nick," announced Rob as they grabbed their bags and headed into the house.

"Trust me, I'm famous to the women I've brought up here," bragged Nick.

"As long as you've got plenty of beer and food, that's all I care about," interjected Zach.

"Don't worry. Barbie and I drove up last weekend, and we stocked the place to the hilt," assured Nick. "We've got enough food and drinks for an army."

"But is that enough for Ryan's last weekend as a free man?," asked Cory. "And who is Barbie? Is that really her name?"

"Barbie is my date for the wedding, and yes, no kidding, it's her name. Anyway, if the food runs out, that's what pizza delivery is for," said Nick. "And there's a liquor store only fifteen minutes away."

The gang swarmed into the house, most of them dumping their bags in the living room and immediately moving out to the deck to pop open a beer and check out the lake. Ryan headed to the back of the house and staked his claim on a bedroom so he wouldn't have to sleep on the floor or the couch, as both had clearly seen better days. "The ultimate bachelor pad for my bachelor party," thought Ryan, looking around the room. The bed was unmade, with sheets and blankets tossed rumpled from the previous occupant. "It must be time for me to get married, since this actually looks unappealing to me," decided Ryan. He tossed his stuff on the bed and went to join his friends.

The long weekend exceeded Ryan's expectations. Everyone got along fine, with only a few exceptions that Ryan wrote off to irritable attitudes from morning hangovers. The guys cruised the lake on Nick's boat and jet skis, drinking, eating, and repeating old stories of their high school glory days, their accomplishments embellished more with every telling. True to form, Nick brought in a few strippers on Saturday night, but Ryan wasn't even tempted to stray. He enjoyed hanging out with his old buddies, but now that the weekend was over, more than anything Ryan was looking forward to his honeymoon the next week.

Elise and Ryan had splurged on an amazing trip to the Virgin Islands, where they planned to scuba dive, sail, relax, and escape from the craziness of their overblown wedding. "Why is it that weddings always seem to take on a life of their own?," thought Ryan. Their guest list had doubled from their original plan. Ryan realized, though, that Elise had much more on her plate as the bride than he had to deal with as the groom. "All I've got left to do in these last two days is get all the guys to the final fitting for the tuxedos and figure out a schedule to pick up friends and relatives from the airport."

Ryan shifted uncomfortably in his car seat as he headed across town toward the tuxedo rental store. He realized he'd been scratching at his crotch off and on for the last day or so, although it wasn't bothering him now nearly as much as it did during the night. The night before, Ryan had woken up multiple times clawing at his pubic area from an intense itch, but when the irritation faded in the morning, Ryan had completely forgotten about it. He reached under the seatbelt for a better angle to scratch. Now that he was conscious of it again, Ryan was worried. "I hope I'm not getting poison ivy again," he fretted.

Last summer, Ryan had had such a bad case of poison ivy that the rash and itch came and went for almost six weeks. He had required two separate rounds of steroid pill packs and one shot of additional steroids. They had not initially realized that his roommate's dog, Corby, was the source, constantly reexposing Ryan. They had eventually learned that the irritants from poison ivy stay on animal fur, and once they quit letting Corby run through the bushes at the park, Ryan's rash finally cleared up.

The last thing Ryan wanted to deal with during his honeymoon was an itchy rash in his groin that he knew would only get worse with sun exposure and heat. Ryan spotted an urgent care clinic and pulled into the parking lot, thinking he could pop in, get a quick steroid shot, and avoid a severe reaction. Looking at his watch, Ryan felt that he had plenty of time before he needed to be at the tuxedo rental place. He considered calling his regular doctor, but even if Dr. Kubiak agreed to call in some medicine, Ryan felt like he would respond more quickly if he could get an injection. He entered the clinic and checked in.

Before long, Ryan was following a young lady down the hallway, where she weighed him and chatted pleasantly while taking his vital signs and guiding him into an exam room. "I'm Susan, Dr. Wright's medical assistant. What seems to be bothering you today?"

"Well, I was at the lake last weekend, and I think perhaps I'm getting poison ivy," explained Ryan. "I'm actually getting married this weekend..."

"Congratulations," Susan chirped.

"Thanks. Anyway, we're headed to the Virgin Islands..."

"Lucky dogs," she interjected.

"Uh, yeah. But I don't want to head down there with poison ivy," Ryan finished quickly. "Do you think I can get a steroid shot?"

"I don't see why not," Susan answered. "We give them all the time for poison ivy, and we've been seeing a bunch of it lately. We'll see what Dr. Wright says in a few minutes when he comes in. Where is your rash?"

"In my crotch, I guess. To be honest, I haven't even looked to see if there's a rash. It feels pretty much like when I had poison ivy last year though. I don't live in town anymore, so when I saw your clinic, I thought it would be best to come in and treat this as soon as possible."

"Fair enough," Susan agreed. "Why don't you change into this gown, with your underwear off please, so Dr. Wright can examine you? We'll get you all fixed up for your wedding."

"Okay," said Ryan, reaching for the gown. Once Susan left, Ryan undressed and put on the gown, hoping he had guessed correctly by having it open to the back, like a hospital gown. He looked at his groin and saw only one bright red, raised line toward the edge of his pubic hair. "Good," he thought. "It doesn't look too bad yet." The rash last year had covered his groin, belly, back, and thighs, plus he had a few marks on his forearms. Ryan sat on the end of the exam table, checking scores, surfing the Internet, and playing games on his phone to kill the time while he waited. Considering how quickly he had been taken into an exam room, it was a long wait for the doctor to arrive. Finally, the door opened and an older gentleman wearing cowboy boots, jeans, a neatly pressed plaid button-down shirt, and a full-length white lab coat entered the room.

"Howdy, I'm Dr. Wright," said the man, extending his hand.

Ryan returned his firm handshake. "Hi, I'm Ryan. Thanks for seeing me."

"Sorry about the wait. We had a few emergencies slip in before you," apologized Dr. Wright.

"If you can fix me by Saturday, it's all good," responded Ryan.

"Oh, that's right," said the doctor. "Susan mentioned you're getting married this weekend. Congratulations. I'll do my best to solve your problem by then, but no promises 'til I see what we're dealing with."

"I think it's poison ivy. It doesn't look that bad yet, but I had a terrible case last year," explained Ryan. "It itches really bad."

"When did you first notice it bothering you?," asked the doctor.

"I think it started yesterday. It definitely was itching last night and this morning."

"Do you know where you might have been exposed?," inquired Dr. Wright.

"My bachelor party was out at the lake last weekend. We hiked through a bunch of weeds when we walked out to my friend's dock, so it could have been there," answered Ryan.

"Bachelor party, eh? Any new sexual partners?," said Dr. Wright.

"No way," replied Ryan, somewhat offended. "Why do you ask?"

"Well, you know what they say, son. If a dog itches, sometimes it's ticks, and sometimes it's fleas."

"What? I'm not following you."

"I simply mean that you could have poison ivy, and you could have caught something else," clarified the doctor. "You would not be the first groom to catch something that made his groin itch from his bachelor party."

"Yeah, but I would be the last. My fiancée would kill me," Ryan tried to joke back. "But seriously, it's not a concern."

"All right, then let's take a look. Go ahead and lay back, son," instructed Dr. Wright, grabbing a pair of gloves out of a box and slipping them on his hands.

Ryan wondered what the doctor was doing when Dr. Wright grabbed the otoscope off the wall. "Isn't that to look in ears?," Ryan asked.

"Yes, but it's also a great lighted magnifying glass," clarified the doctor.

Dr. Wright lifted Ryan's patient gown and quickly focused on the red streak Ryan had noticed earlier. "This is an irritated scratch right here, but there are no blisters or clear discharge or anything suggestive of poison ivy," commented Dr. Wright. He continued to look around Ryan's thighs and pubic region until something else caught his attention. "Bingo!," he exclaimed.

"What?," asked Ryan, rising up on his elbows.

"Unfortunately, son, you have indeed picked up a crawling critter, but not ticks or fleas," Dr. Wright declared. "You've got crabs."

"Crabs? No way. I told you, I didn't have sex with anybody. I swear it," Ryan argued defensively.

"Where did you sleep last weekend?," inquired the doctor.

Ryan closed his eyes and let his head drop forward, shaking it back and forth. "In my friend's disgusting bachelor pad," he admitted.

"I'm guessing the sheets were less than clean, then," responded Dr. Wright.

"Apparently," confirmed Ryan.

"Well, the good news is that it's not poison ivy, so you don't need steroids. The bad news is that this is extremely contagious. You've got to be sure that you and all of your clothing and bedding are completely treated, so you don't give this to your bride this weekend. That most certainly would not be a welcome wedding gift."

"Will it be gone by this weekend?," asked Ryan nervously.

"Well, the medicine kills off any adult lice, but if you don't remove all of the eggs, which are called nits, then they could hatch next week on your honeymoon."

"How do I get rid of the eggs?"

"You can use a fine-toothed comb. They usually sell special combs along with the medicated shampoos that kill the lice," responded Dr. Wright.

"And you said I need to treat my clothes and bedding too? How do I do that?," inquired Ryan.

"Everything that can be put in the washing machine should be washed in hot water with detergent and then dried in the dryer for at least twenty minutes. Anything that can't be washed needs to be put in an airtight plastic bag and sealed off for ten to fourteen days. There are also medicated sprays that you can spray on couches and chairs," explained the doctor.

Ryan was going through everything in his head, realizing he would have to make time to wash all of his clothes that were back at the hotel. A trip to a laundromat was now added to his to-do list. Suddenly it seemed that the clock was ticking too fast, with extra tasks cropping up left and right. "Okay, so where do I get the medicine? Is it prescription?," he asked.

"No, there are a couple of brands that you can buy over the counter," replied Dr. Wright. "We generally don't use the prescription type unless the other ones don't seem to work, because the prescription one has more potential side effects. My nurse will give you a handout with the names of all the available products, as well as printed instructions for treating your clothes and bedding. You should be able to pick up everything across the street at the pharmacy or grocery store. If I were you, I'd pick up a second treatment to take with you on your honeymoon just in case anything else crops up, although usually one application will take care of it. Any other questions?," asked Dr. Wright.

"I don't think so," said Ryan thoughtfully. "I really need to get rid of these, uh, crabs as fast as possible. My fiancée will be pretty freaked out when she finds out about this problem. Luckily, we've barely seen each other this week."

"Have you shared a bed with her, or any other spot, since your party?," asked the doctor.

"No, we haven't," Ryan answered happily.

"Great, then she shouldn't have been exposed. My best wishes to the bride," smiled Dr. Wright, "and good luck to you."

Ryan got dressed, paid the bill at the front desk, and double-checked that he had the treatment instructions as he got into his car. He started the car and checked his watch, trying to decide if he had time to go to the pharmacy across the street before he headed to the tuxedo rental store.

"Oh man," Ryan suddenly agonized, "what are we going to do about the tuxedos?" With everyone at the same house last weekend, it was conceivable that Ryan was not the only one who had acquired crabs. And now, they were all supposed to go and try on rental tuxedos. Didn't the doctor tell him that crabs could be spread through clothing? Gross. Ryan didn't want to be responsible for spreading this infection around. They would simply all have to get treated before they could go to the tuxedo shop. "They are never, ever going to let me live this down," Ryan thought.

He dialed information on his cell phone and soon was connected with the shop. "Hi, this is Ryan..."

"Ryan Anderson?," asked the salesman at the store.

"Yes, that's me," replied Ryan.

"Great. Two of your groomsmen have arrived here ahead of you, and we can get started on their measurements, but we'll obviously need you here for your final fitting as well. Are you far away?," asked the man.

"Actually, uh, something's come up. I... I can't make it there today," stammered Ryan. "Will it be a problem if we all show up first thing tomorrow?"

"Well," snipped the salesman with some irritation, "I can't promise we'll still have everything, but we'll make do. Can you be here promptly at ten in the morning when we open?"

Ryan breathed a sigh of relief. "Yes, ten is no problem. Thank you. Can you ask my friends to call me?"

"So you can tell them what 'came up'?"

"Yeah. Sorry again," said Ryan as he ended the call.

Within seconds, his phone was ringing. "Ryan?," said Nick. "What's up? I thought Elise said we had to get this done today. You know, she's going to blame me if we don't get the right penguin suits."

Ryan practically bit his tongue. "Oh, Elise is going to blame you, all right," he retorted. "Nick, do me a favor and step outside the rental shop. I don't want you to repeat out loud what I'm going to tell you."

"What are you talking about? The guy says he can take our measurements while we're here," Nick responded.

"Seriously. Please tell him you'll be back in the morning. Come on, Nick, don't mess around. Please just step outside," Ryan begged.

"Okay, okay, I'm outside, but Ben is still in there. What is so important?," Nick asked impatiently.

"Nick, I got crabs from your love shack last weekend," accused Ryan.

"Crabs? Isn't that pubic lice? Ha! Are you kidding me? I think you're being paranoid," Nick assessed.

"Trust me. I walked out of the doctor's office a minute ago. The guy found crab eggs in my crotch," rebutted Ryan.

"There's no way, Ryan. How could you get that from my lake house? If you did, it was from those strippers. Dude, I thought you stayed pretty much out of their way," said Nick, laughing through the phone.

"Nick, it's not funny. I got them from the sheets, and you slept there the weekend before, so I'd bet you have them too. For that matter, I think we probably all need to get treated before we put on rented suits and spread this around even more. Meet me at my hotel, and I'll pick up the medicine for everyone at the pharmacy."

"Okay, Mr. Responsible, but I think you're going overboard," replied Nick.

"By the way, I'd rather that Elise and the other women not know about this," Ryan suggested.

"So they won't get crabby?," teased Nick.

Ryan rolled his eyes. With these guys, he'd be lucky if lice didn't become the main theme of the weekend. How would his in-laws-to-be react if they found out? What a hassle. "Whatever, Nick. Go ahead, get it out of your system, and make all the jokes you want with me today. I'm seriously asking you, as my best man, to help me put this to rest so it doesn't ruin the wedding weekend for Elise. See you at the hotel, okay?"

"Gotcha." Nick chuckled and, true to his nature, couldn't resist adding, "We'll bug out of here right now. Don't worry, I'll think of an excuse that's not too... lousy."

Ryan shook his head, but he had to laugh at the bad puns. Nick's quick wit had earned him a reputation as the class clown growing up, always keeping the gang laughing. Ryan hoped he could convince Nick to resist the temptation to talk about crabs during his best-man toast at the wedding.

facts

Pubic Lice Fact Sheet

What is it?

- "Crabs" is the common name for pubic lice. The scientific name for this tiny, 1.2 mm, six-legged parasitic insect is Phthirus pubis.
- A medical name for the infestation is pediculosis.

How common is it?

- Pubic lice infestation is common worldwide.
- The National Institute of Allergy and Infectious Diseases estimates that 3 million people are newly infected in the United States each year.
- The incidence rate of pubic lice is 1 in 90 people in the United States.

How do you get it?

- Crabs are transmitted most often through intercourse but also by direct contact with infected bed linens, clothing, or towels.

- People trying on bathing suits at stores without wearing underwear can transmit or pick up pubic lice.

Where on your body do you get it?

- Pubic lice primarily infest pubic hair.

- They can also infest armpit hair, eyebrows, eyelashes, mustaches, and beards.

How do I know if I have it?

- Pubic lice cause moderate to severe itching, which is typically worse at night.

- Close inspection of pubic hair reveals small white or yellow oval dots, usually fixed near the base of the hair shaft. These are nits, the eggs of the lice.

- Adult lice can often be found in the seams of clothing.

What does it look like?

- The creature itself has a round body with six legs. The front two legs are larger, closely resembling the pincer claws of a crab when looked at under magnification. Adults are tan to grayish-white.

- Small white dots on pubic hairs can be seen with the naked eye.

- Because the itching leads to scratching, most people have scratch marks, called excoriations, around the pubic region.

- Sometimes the bites will cause a bluish-gray reaction in the skin.
- Scratching and thus opening the skin can cause secondary bacterial infections, which are called impetigos.

What does it feel like?

- Pubic lice need human blood to survive, so they bury their heads in the pubic hair follicle, excreting an irritating substance into the skin that causes moderate to severe itching.

How long does it last?

- Pubic lice last until the person is treated with appropriate medicine and the environmental infestation is eliminated (to avoid reinfestation).
- Each female adult louse lays 30 to 50 eggs during her life span.
- If an infestation is many adults, symptoms can begin immediately.
- If an infestation is only a few adults, symptoms may not be obvious for 2–4 weeks as the adults lay eggs. The eggs take over a week to hatch, mature, and proliferate.

Can it be cured?

- Yes, but the environment must be treated as well to prevent reinfestation.

Can you be reinfected?

- Yes, you can be reinfected.

What is the treatment?

- Over-the-counter medicines contain permethrin or permethrin with piperonyl butoxide, both of which kill only adult lice.
- Prescription washes contain hexachlorocyclohexane, also known as lindane, which must be used with caution due to potential nervous system side effects. Only a physician or other authorized prescribing medical personnel should decide whether this is the correct treatment for your lice.
- Over-the-counter medicated shampoos are applied to dry pubic hair, worked in for 5–10 minutes, and thoroughly rinsed. Remaining nits should then be removed with a fine-toothed comb.
- Usually a single treatment is all that is needed, but some infestations require a second treatment 5–10 days later (to remove the nymph and adult stages of lice that may have hatched from any remaining nits).
- For eyelash infestations, only petroleum jelly can be used (to smother the lice). No shampoo, cream, or ointment containing anti-lice medications should ever be used on the eyes.
- Bedding and clothing must be washed in hot water and dried in a hot dryer for at least 20 minutes.
- Items that cannot be washed must be sprayed with a medicated spray or sealed in plastic bags for 10–14 days to suffocate the lice.
- All intimate contacts—including not only sexual partners, but anyone who has shared bedding, towels, or clothing—and their environments should be treated at the same time.

How about alternative therapies?

- Occlusive dressings, such as petroleum jelly or mayonnaise, have limited effectiveness and are not recommended for the pubic area, although petroleum jelly is used for infestations of the eyelashes.

- Shaving is not necessary to treat lice infestation and does not prevent infection.

Are there long-term consequences?

- Lice infestation by itself does not lead to long-term problems.

- Secondary infections from repeated scratching could rarely cause further complications or scarring.

When are you contagious?

- If you are infected, you are contagious until you and your environment are fully treated.

- Pubic lice are thought to be potentially the most infectious STI.

- One contact with an infected partner results in a 95% chance of transmission.

- Condoms do not reduce the transmission of pubic lice, because they do not cover pubic hair.

Can crabs be transmitted between homosexual partners?

- Absolutely.

How do I avoid catching crabs?

- Abstain from intercourse and direct genital contact with new partners (and their bedding).
- Avoid contact with other people's used sheets; don't sleep in others' bedding.
- Wear underwear when trying on swimsuits or undergarments in stores.

If I have crabs, how do I avoid giving it to my partner?

- Meticulously follow the medication instructions to rid your body, your clothing, and your linens of the pubic lice, and do not have intimate contact for 10 days after initial treatment.
- If you have been intimate with any partners during your infestation, they need to treat themselves and their environment as well, to avoid passing the lice back and forth.

Frequently Asked Questions

➤ **Do you have to have sex to catch crabs?**
No. Pubic lice can be transmitted from close genital contact or through infested bed linens, clothing, or towels.

➤ **Did I catch crabs from a toilet seat?**
Very unlikely. Pubic lice don't live long off humans and don't have the capacity to grip smooth surfaces, such as a toilet seat.

➤ **Did I get crabs from oral sex?**
Unlikely. Potentially, you could get a pubic lice infestation on your eyelashes or facial hair from performing oral sex.

➤ **Are pubic lice the same as head lice?**
No. Pubic lice are not found on the scalp. They can be

distinguished under the microscope by their body type: pubic lice are short and round, whereas head lice are longer and oval. Treatment, however, is similar.

➤ **Are pubic lice the same thing as scabies?**
No, but they are very similar. Both are infestations that are easily transmitted sexually or less commonly via contaminated linens. However, scabies is caused by a mite that burrows underneath the skin anywhere on the body, often in the genital area, especially on men. Scabies infections may take up to two months before they cause symptoms. The symptoms of a scabies infestation are the same as the symptoms of pubic lice: itching, often worse at night. People with weakened immune systems (such as in advanced HIV disease) may develop a severe form of scabies called "crusted scabies," which can affect the entire body, including the nails and hair, and therefore this type may be confused with other skin conditions, such as psoriasis. Household members and any sexual contacts during the previous month should all be treated for scabies, and all linens and clothing should be decontaminated in the same manner as is done for pubic lice infestations. Treatment is prescription scabicide lotion or cream (lindane, crotamiton, or permethrin).

➤ **Did I catch this from trying on swimsuits?**
Possibly. Always wear underwear when trying on swimsuits or undergarments to decrease (although not eliminate) chances of getting this infestation.

➤ **Did I get this from my dog or cat?**
No. Pubic lice cannot live on or be transmitted by animals, only humans.

Additional Information

American Sexual Health Association
PO Box 13827
Research Triangle Park, NC 27709

919-361-8400
www.ashasexualhealth.org/

Centers for Disease Control and Prevention
1600 Clifton Road
Atlanta, GA 30329-4027
1-800-CDC-INFO (1-800-232-4636), 1-888-232-6348 (TTY)
www.cdc.gov/ncidod/dpd/parasites/lice/factsht_pubic_lice.htm

MedlinePlus
US National Library of Medicine
8600 Rockville Pike
Bethesda, MD 20894
1-888-FIND-NLM (1-888-346-3656) or 301-594-5983
www.nlm.nih.gov/medlineplus/ency/article/000841.htm

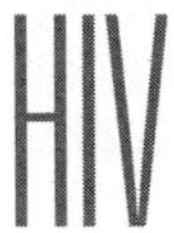

15: Evan

EVAN WALKED IN THE door after work, exhausted from standing on his feet all afternoon. For Christmas break, he had returned to his old summer job as a grocery checker. Being back at home was a mixed blessing. Evan hated having to follow someone else's schedule, but it was wonderful to come home to delicious home-cooked meals instead of the slop that passed for food back at the college cafeteria. Tonight he smelled his favorite—good old spaghetti and meatballs.

"Oh good, you're back in time for dinner. We're just sitting down to eat. Come join us after you wash your hands," his mom said.

Evan managed to wash his hands without making any smart-aleck comments about being old enough to know to do this without his mother's advice, and then sat down to eat. He would be headed back to school and those fast food dinners in a few days, so he knew he'd better savor this meal.

"By the way, the doctor's office called today saying they couldn't reach you, and Dr. Litz wants you to come in tomorrow to discuss your lab work from your physical this week. I made an appointment for you at eight fifteen tomorrow morning, so it won't interfere with your work schedule. I hope everything's okay." The last comment was more of a question than a statement. Evan shrugged as he grabbed some butter to slather on his second roll.

"I'm sure it's no big deal, Mom. Didn't they have anything later in the morning? Faith and I are going to a late movie tonight."

"You're headed back out?"

"Don't even go there, honey," Evan's dad said to his wife, placing his hand on her arm. "Take a cab if you two have anything to drink, son."

Evan rolled his eyes and said, "Dad, you know I'm underage. We're going to a movie, not bar hopping on Sixth Street." The rest of the meal was fairly quiet, with Evan finishing off a third plate of spaghetti and meatballs while his mom discreetly tried to pump him for information about his new girlfriend.

His parents had been less than thrilled last semester when they realized that his first girlfriend in college—actually, his first serious girlfriend ever—was not only six years older than him but had already been married and divorced. Evan had never been particularly impressed with girls his age in high school. They were always obsessed with superficial things like fashion, reality television shows, and gossip. Courtney had been the first woman who ever shared his passions about more important things, like social justice and politics, and she also happened to share his taste in music. Courtney had asked him out to hear a local band after work one night, and he had quickly fallen for her. When Evan later found out that she was still involved sporadically with her ex-husband, he was heartbroken. He stayed with Courtney for a couple of months but finally broke up with her when he realized that she seemed incapable of making a clean break from her ex.

But there was no threat of any unfinished business with his new girlfriend, Faith. She was one year younger than Evan, still in high school, and was a virgin when they began dating a few weeks ago. Evan had really enjoyed the sexual intimacy that Courtney had taught him, and he quickly became sexually active with Faith. Faith was already on the pill to control her painful periods, but Evan made sure to use condoms to protect against disease as well. He knew he should have been more consistent about using condoms with Courtney, but he was going to be sure that he and Faith were completely safe.

The next morning, his alarm jarred him from sleep. He grabbed a clean T-shirt and jeans from his laundry basket; his mom must have washed his clothes for him the night before. As he drove to Dr. Litz's office, Evan wondered what was so important that she wanted to bring him in to discuss his bloodwork. He had had his annual physical with her a couple of days earlier in the week. He had agreed to STI testing after admitting that he had not always been perfect about wearing a condom. Could it be gonorrhea or something? He had absolutely no symptoms. Maybe his blood count was low again. A couple of years ago he had been vegetarian for a year and had become a little anemic. Not much chance of that this year. He laughed about how much he had enjoyed his mother's meatballs.

Evan checked in with the receptionist, showed his insurance card for the second time in three days, and forked over his ten dollar co-pay. He went through the motions of being weighed and getting his temperature and blood pressure taken, and practically fell asleep while he sat in the chair waiting for the doctor. Dr. Litz actually came in pretty quickly, but she didn't seem to be her usual joking self. Evan sat up, his heart suddenly racing. "What's up?," he asked.

"Evan, I've known you since you were a little boy. You know that I always tell you the truth. Well, now I've got some news, and it's scary, but I'm going to tell you everything, and we'll get through it, okay?" Dr. Litz was looking him straight in the eye and had put her hand on his knee as she pulled her rolling stool right in front of him. Evan was wide awake now and felt vaguely nauseated as his heart pounded practically out of his chest.

"What? What is it?," he demanded.

"You know we tested you for all the usual bloodwork plus STIs. Well, everything else came back normal, but your HIV test came back positive."

"HIV? Oh my God, HIV? I'm nineteen years old—I haven't even picked a major yet!" Evan's thoughts raced. He realized Dr. Litz had stopped talking and was waiting for him to open his eyes and look at her.

She slowed down her speech and made sure he was focused on her. "I want you to really listen to what I'm saying. At this point, this only means that you have a positive test for HIV. It hopefully will prove to be a false positive, but we've got to do more tests to figure that out. The frustrating part is that those confirmatory tests take several days to get results, so you'll be in limbo wondering whether or not this is real. In the meantime, here's the bottom line. This HIV test that you took is designed to catch as many true positives as possible. Because of that, if you are in a low-risk population, the chance of a positive result being a false positive can be up to fifty percent. However, if you are in a high-risk group, then the likelihood of it being a true positive is actually very high. Our job right now is to go back over your history, and let's figure out if you are truly high or low risk, okay?"

Evan's brain was still spinning, but he nodded in agreement. He hadn't quite found his voice yet. Dr. Litz continued, "Now, Evan, I've got to ask you several questions that I should already know the answers to, but we need to be thorough. Have you ever used any IV drugs?"

"Yeah, right." He rolled his eyes. "No, never," he said, seeing in Dr. Litz's expression that this was no time for sarcasm.

"Have you ever had any sexual activity with another guy?," she asked. This time, he gave a simple no.

"Okay, your first girlfriend that you had sex with—what was her name?"

"Courtney."

"That's right, Courtney. Now, as I recall, she was previously married, right?," the doctor asked.

"Yes."

"Do you happen to know if she had any other partners before her husband?"

"Yeah. She had one other high school boyfriend before James," Evan replied.

"Do we have any idea if that high school boyfriend had previous partners?"

"Not a clue."

"Okay, then, back to James, the ex-husband. What do we know about him?," Dr. Litz asked.

"That he's a jerk. And an addict," Evan snorted.

Dr. Litz's heart sank, but she tried to keep her voice steady. "What kind of addict? Did he use IV drugs?"

Evan shrugged. "I have no idea. Courtney referred to him as being an addict. I kind of assumed she meant pot or cocaine or something, but now I'm not so sure. It never seemed important to ask."

"What about his sexual history?," asked the doctor.

Evan thought for a minute. "Well, I do know that he already has a new girlfriend, because they were apparently sleeping together while Courtney and I were together. It turned out that Courtney was still occasionally sleeping with James, which is why we broke up."

"And the girlfriend? Do we have any clue?"

"No. But she's even older, like thirty, and I do know she has kids, so obviously she's had at least one other partner," Evan muttered.

Dr. Litz paused, then asked, "Did you have any discussions with Courtney about whether or not she'd had an STI or STI testing before?"

Evan thought for a minute, then replied, "You know, actually, she did get something from James once, but she commented that thank goodness one round of antibiotics cured whatever it was. In fact, that's how she found out originally that he was cheating on her when they were married."

"So, it sounds like James probably has had several partners," the doctor said quietly.

"Oh man, I never thought about it that way before..." Evan sank his head into his hands and rubbed his temples. "I'll bet he's had dozens of partners. Crap, why on earth didn't I think about this before? Dr. Litz, it's not fair, I'm *not* that way, and here I'm the one with... with a positive test." Evan couldn't bring himself to even say "HIV" yet.

Dr. Litz sadly shook her head and sighed. "You're absolutely right, Evan, it isn't fair. You feel like you've only had sex with one person before your current girlfriend, but the truth is that you effectively sleep not just with that person, but with everyone that person has slept with, and so on and so on. Even if Courtney had only slept with two men, and each of them had slept with two other women, that would expose you to at least six other people just by having sex with Courtney."

Evan interrupted. "And you can bet that James slept with a heck of a lot more than two women, and I highly doubt their virginity... All of which means I'm screwed, doesn't it? Does this make me high risk?"

Again, Dr. Litz shook her head. "Honestly, I'm not sure. We used to define high risk as anyone who had over six partners when it came to STIs. You can do the math that with six direct contacts, you're quickly into some very high numbers for exposure. The biggest problem here is that we're not sure about your secondary exposure. However, we do know that you don't have any of the other big risk factors—drug use or homosexual contact—so overall, I still think that there is a solid chance that this will turn out to be a false positive."

"So back to that false positive thing. Why would you use a test that can come back as a false positive half the time? That doesn't make any sense to me," said Evan.

"No, no, that's not what I meant. A false positive actually occurs only once in about three hundred thousand tests. In an isolated test, when there is a positive test result, if that person is truly low risk, that specific test has up to a fifty percent false positive rate. Does that make sense?"

"Um, no."

"Okay, let me give you an example. If you take a healthy, non-smoking, thirty-something female runner and give her a stress treadmill test to look for heart disease, there is an extremely low chance of it being positive. Because of that, if it *is* positive, it's more likely to be a false positive than a true positive because she has no risk factors for heart disease. Does that make more sense to you?"

"Yeah, actually, it does. So I either have HIV, or I'm the 'lucky winner' of a one in three hundred thousand chance of having a false positive. Great," Evan said sarcastically.

"Or, let's say that you still have up to a fifty-fifty chance that it's not real. Let's leave the glass half full, okay?," smiled Dr. Litz.

"Easy for you to say. It's looking half empty from here. So what if it is real? Then what happens next?," he asked.

"Well, we get you right in with an infectious disease specialist, and they will decide about starting you on antiviral drugs."

She thought for a minute, and then added, "Evan, do you know the difference between having HIV and having AIDS?"

"No, I really don't. Aren't they the same?"

"Not at all. Many people are HIV-positive but continue functioning perfectly well for years. It's not until the HIV has attacked and killed off most of the body's immune defenses that people develop the opportunistic infections that are diagnostic of AIDS. There are skin and respiratory infections that cannot take place in a healthy immune system and occur only when those defenses are shut down. When a person gets these specific infections, then they receive the diagnosis of AIDS."

"Okay, assuming I'm positive, Dr. Litz, how long am I going to live?" Evan took a deep breath and really focused on the doctor.

"Evan, I don't have a crystal ball, but right now the time from the diagnosis of HIV-positive antibodies until the onset of AIDS can be many years—up to a normal life span. We used to feel getting HIV was a death sentence, but now many people are leading productive lives and dealing with their HIV disease much like others deal with diabetes or any other chronic illness. I'm confident we'll continue to advance our research and improve our drugs, fighting both HIV itself and the infections that take over when the immune system is beaten down. In fact, we can no longer predict the average life expectancy even from the diagnosis of AIDS because every year the numbers are improving."

Dr. Litz continued, "You might be wondering why in the heck I am telling you about this test before we know for sure one way or another. The biggest reason is that you told me this week that you are sleeping with a new girlfriend. Ethically, I absolutely had to tell you in order to minimize her risk. You don't get or give HIV from hugging, kissing, or sharing food, but you certainly can transmit it by sex. I'm glad you've been using condoms, but condoms can break, and if you are HIV-positive, your new girlfriend needs to know. I know this is a ton to digest, but do you have any questions right now?"

"How long until we know for sure?"

"Hopefully less than a week. Our lab sends your blood to California to run the Western blot test, which is a DNA test that takes several days to process. We'll also draw your blood again today for another test to check for the amount of virus in your blood, and that test should actually be back in a few days," she replied.

"So if the quicker test is negative?"

"That's great news, but we still wait for the Western blot DNA test to be one hundred percent sure," she replied.

Evan's brain was still racing; mainly he was furious with Courtney and wondering how quickly he could reach her by phone to grill her about her ex. Evan couldn't bear to think about Faith. He could picture her beautiful innocent eyes filling with tears when he told her the news. Man, he would kill Courtney if this turned out to really be HIV. One in three hundred thousand . . . could he really be that unlucky? Of course, at this point, it would actually be lucky for it to turn out to be a false positive. If only there were a way to really know his risk.

Dr. Litz's voice interrupted his thoughts. "Evan?" He looked up.

Dr. Litz smiled reassuringly. "Either way, we'll get through this." She handed him her business card. "Here are the best ways to reach me. I'm sure you'll have more questions later, so feel free to call whenever. Is your cell phone the best way to reach you?"

"Absolutely. Please don't call my parents' home. They would totally freak out. I'm not going to tell them until we know for certain, okay?," he pleaded.

"Evan, don't worry. You're nineteen. Anything we discuss stays between us unless you ask me to tell them something. But you know, if you do want me to talk to your parents, I'd be happy to do so."

"Not now. Let's wait and see what the tests show. So, you'll call as soon as you hear?"

"I promise. The minute we receive the results, I'll call you on your cell. I know how anxious you'll be. Let's try to stay optimistic, and I'll talk to you later this week. Okay?" Dr. Litz hoped her voice didn't reflect her true suspicions. The reality was that with Evan's secondary contacts, it sounded like he was not in the low-risk category, which meant that his Western blot test was likely to come back confirming HIV disease.

Evan took his lab slip and other paperwork from Dr. Litz. What a morning this had been. His hand gripped tightly the cell phone in his pocket. He checked out and walked around the corner toward the lab. Before he went in to get his blood drawn, he stopped and leaned against the wall, feeling almost faint for a moment. He pulled out his phone to text Courtney, but as the magnitude of the whole thing began to really hit him, he simply sank down to the floor and sat, head in his hands. It was all too much.

16: Tanya

TANYA SMILED AT HER reflection in the mirror as she removed the extra earrings from her upper ears. Looking back at her was a polished, professional woman. Her long hair was slicked back in a tidy French knot, revealing only tasteful diamond studs in her earlobes. Tanya plucked a few cat hairs off the shoulder of her stylish navy blue suit. "I can't have animal fur messing up this perfect picture," she giggled.

Since she was old enough to remember, Tanya had taken in every stray or wounded animal that she found. From fallen baby birds to lost dogs or cats, Tanya loved to nurse them back to health and find new homes for them. Tanya's mom, an animal lover herself, supported Tanya's actions, but she set a rule that any animal brought in the house had a two-week grace period during which Tanya must find it a permanent home. As Tanya looked around her apartment at Sir Lance, her cat; Calypso, her parakeet; a tank full of fish; and her old dog, Shadow, she could see the wisdom in that rule.

Tanya thought wistfully of her mother. "If only you could see me now, Mom," she mused. "I look so conservative, you'd think I vote Republican." Her mom had died, still worrying about Tanya's future, before Tanya had finished college. If she could only see her former "wild child" starting a job as a full-fledged certified public accountant, she would be at peace.

Tanya had rebelled during her first couple of years in college.

"Your friends look like the strays that we've always taken in," her mother had commented more than once. Tanya would immediately defend her companions. "Mom, their clothes are vintage, and you should be impressed that they shop at thrift stores rather than spending a ton of money on high-end fashion."

Her father's words were significantly harsher. "Tanya, you'll be judged by the company you keep. Young people dressed head to toe in black and smoking cigarettes don't impress anyone, and you befriending these drug addicts isn't noble—it's stupid. Don't call me to bail you out of jail."

"They're not drug addicts," Tanya had protested, but in truth, the crowd she hung out with not only partied hard with alcohol and cigarettes, but most smoked pot and many of them routinely experimented with other drugs "to help get their creative juices flowing."

Over half of the group was involved in theater, and they carried their flair for the dramatic off the stage and into their everyday life. Constant political and social debates challenged many of Tanya's childhood beliefs. Late-night arguments about the need to legalize marijuana offered Tanya new perspectives on what had previously been a black-and-white issue to her. Perhaps the most startling behavior to Tanya was the group's acceptance of casual sex partners, which they referred to as "friends with benefits."

Tanya began to experiment with her appearance, adding several ear piercings and a belly-button ring, reveling in the freedom of this self-expression. Eventually she even got a small tattoo of a dove but placed it in an easily concealed location over her right shoulder blade. Her family worried about her external changes, fearing that she was headed down a path of self-destruction. However, while Tanya's ideas had liberalized a bit, her actions remained very conservative within this social group, and she never indulged beyond a couple of beers or a glass of wine.

Tanya's thoughts turned briefly to Devon, her first serious boyfriend and the dominant personality in the group. Devon had grown up traveling around the world with his father's oil business. Tall and slender, with thick jet-black hair and a vaguely British accent, Devon had enchanted Tanya from the moment they met. She was fascinated with his sophisticated ideas and zest for life. Tanya dated him exclusively for nearly two years, despite the fact that he openly continued to see other women. Tanya had naively thought that if she could make him love her enough, he wouldn't need others to satisfy his desires. After giving up her virginity, her emotional innocence, and two years of her life, Tanya moved on to more mutually beneficial relationships during the rest of college.

Today, Tanya was decidedly happy to be single. It had taken all of her time and energy throughout the last year to study for and pass the CPA exam, and she was excited about her first real day of work. The last few weeks had been considered orientation to the firm, covering all different areas of accounting as well as explanations of her benefits, from retirement plans to health and life insurance policies. This morning Tanya would finally start in the audit section, her main area of interest. She gave Shadow a pat on his head, freshened up the water bowls, fed the fish, and headed out the door.

Tanya looked around as she slid through the revolving door at the entrance of her building. "No matter how you slice it, I'm definitely grown up now," she thought, as she headed toward the elevator bank.

"Hey, Tanya," said a deep voice behind her.

"Good morning, Seth," Tanya replied with pleasure. Seth had made it a point to sit next to her during orientation the week before. His new suit complemented his tall, athletic frame. "Nice threads," Tanya added coyly.

"You clean up pretty well yourself." Seth smiled. "Are you nervous about getting started today?"

"Does it show?" Tanya laughed.

"Actually, no, that's why I asked," replied Seth. "I was hoping I wasn't the only one worked up over finally getting started."

"Well, I'm ready, nervous or not. At least now I'll be doing what interests me, instead of all that tax stuff we had to suffer through last week," said Tanya.

"So how about if you and I grab dinner and drinks tonight to celebrate the end of our first real day?," Seth smoothly asked.

Tanya paused for a moment, shouting inside her head, "Sweet!" but out loud saying, "You know, that would be great. Where should we meet?"

"How about here in the lobby at five ten?," suggested Seth, as they entered the elevator together.

"Five ten it is," agreed Tanya, noting to herself that only two accountants would pick such a specific time.

Tanya was deeply engrossed in her work late in the morning when she received a concerning email from human resources.

> Due to abnormal blood test results, additional evaluation is required before we can execute your life insurance policy. Please schedule a follow-up appointment with Health Partners, Inc., as soon as possible.

"Well, that's odd," mused Tanya. "I feel perfectly fine. Bet my cholesterol was high. I should have been watching my diet better before my test." She clicked on the hyperlink for Health Partners and decided she'd call and schedule an appointment before she delved back into her work.

"Health Partners, how may I help you?," answered a receptionist.

"Hi, this is Tanya Leslie, and I'm a new employee at Abbott Accounting. I received a note that I apparently had some abnormal bloodwork on my screening tests for my life insurance policy, and that I should call for an appointment."

"Well, you're in luck, because I just had a cancellation for an afternoon appointment today at three. Can you make that? We're right down the street from your firm. Otherwise, our next opening is at the end of the month, on the twenty-ninth."

Tanya realized that today was better than later in the month, when she would be fully involved in her work, so she agreed. "Fine, let's go with today at 3 p.m."

"Great. Please come fifteen minutes early to fill out paperwork, and bring your insurance card."

Tanya hung up the phone, cleared the afternoon appointment with her supervisor, and resumed her work. "Oh great, this looks brilliant," Tanya thought sarcastically. "A few hours into my first day at work, and I'm asking for time off. I'm in perfect health, and now it looks like I'm some slacker."

At exactly two forty-five, Tanya sat in the doctor's office, completing her new patient forms. "When you answer 'no' to all the questions, it doesn't take fifteen minutes to fill these out," she mused. The forms asked about past surgeries, hospitalizations, pregnancies, and past diseases from asthma to sexually transmittable infections. "The only 'yes' I have is a recent tetanus shot, from when a neighborhood cat accidentally scratched me," reflected Tanya. She turned in her forms and was promptly sent to an exam room. Tanya glanced at her watch, pleased that perhaps she would be back to work quickly. Unfortunately, it was almost three thirty when the doctor finally walked into her exam room, wearing a somber expression on his face.

"Tanya Leslie? I'm Dr. Andrews," said the short, balding physician dressed in a dated coat and tie.

"Hello, nice to meet you," replied Tanya, returning his firm handshake.

"I see from your paperwork that you've been relatively healthy," he began.

"The only time I've been sick in the past five years is when I had mononucleosis my sophomore year in college," agreed Tanya.

"Did they do a blood test?," asked the doctor.

"I honestly don't remember," said Tanya. "I had a fever and a sore throat. They said it was not strep throat and that it was likely mono. There were a ton of students on campus with mono that semester."

"And since then, you've been pretty healthy?," asked Dr. Andrews.

"Since I quit hanging around with smokers, I haven't even had a cold," said Tanya. "Why are you asking all this? What did my test show that is making you look so concerned?"

Dr. Andrews's smile faded, and he took a deep breath. "Tanya, there's no good way to tell you this. Your HIV test came back positive, and it's been confirmed with two additional tests. The first test is a screening test, and it is automatically repeated if there is a positive. After two positives, we send off for a second, more definitive, test called a Western blot. All of your tests were positive."

Tanya's mouth dropped open in disbelief. "HIV? Are you telling me I have AIDS? That's impossible."

"No, you do not have AIDS, but you do have HIV disease. The rest of your lab tests look great, though. You're not anemic, and your white blood cell count is strong."

"Wait a second," interrupted Tanya. "What is the difference

between HIV disease and AIDS? Aren't they the same? This doesn't make any sense to me. And I don't feel bad."

"HIV disease means you are infected with the human immunodeficiency virus. AIDS, which stands for acquired immune deficiency syndrome, refers to the very advanced stage of HIV disease, when the immune system is so damaged that it can't fight off many infections," explained the doctor. "It's great that you appear so healthy otherwise. With all the new medicines that we have to fight HIV, I hope you'll stay that way for a long time."

"I'm sorry," Tanya protested, raising both hands, palms out, in front of her. "There has to be a mistake. I've never done IV drugs, and I'm not promiscuous. I've only had sex with a few guys in my entire life, and none of them were gay or bisexual. I'm not sick. Isn't it far more likely that your test is wrong? I simply don't believe this. Please, why don't we draw my blood again today, and if it comes back positive again, then I'll deal with this, okay? I'll bet my blood sample got switched with someone else's in the lab or something."

"I have to tell you that I do believe these test results are accurate, but certainly we can repeat the test today. I know that this is a lot to absorb, and I've got no doubt that you are a clean-cut young lady. Unfortunately, having sex with anyone, even one man, is a risk, because you don't know for certain his entire past sexual history. HIV disease is not restricted to homosexuals, prostitutes, or IV drug users," lectured Dr. Andrews. "What did you use for protection?"

"I was on the pill," replied Tanya.

"So you didn't think you needed to use condoms?," he asked.

Tanya bit her lip, shaking her head in the negative, and firmly refusing to believe that she could have contracted HIV. "No, it's impossible," she decided, "but if I did, it would have to be Devon, Mr. I-Can't-Limit-Myself-to-One-Person. When was the last time I heard anything about him? John had definitely been a virgin, and Garrett had only a couple of old girlfriends, so it had to be Devon..." Tanya's thoughts raced on, but she realized the doctor had been talking and seemed to be waiting for an answer. "I'm sorry, could you repeat that?," she mumbled apologetically.

"I was saying that if this test confirms the others, we'll get you an appointment with Dr. Fagerberg, an infectious disease specialist.

There are so many new drug protocols that I generally leave it up to the specialist to establish your drug regimen. Do you have any other questions for me right now?," asked Dr. Andrews.

"HIV can't be spread by kissing someone, right?," inquired Tanya.

"Correct. HIV is only spread through direct contact with the blood or body fluids from an infected person, such as through oral, vaginal, or anal sex, or by sharing needles. Casual contact like hugging and kissing does not transmit the virus."

Dr. Andrews examined Tanya, looking in her mouth, eyes, and ears, feeling her neck, and listening to her heart and lungs. "Everything looks good," he reassured her. "Let's recheck your bloodwork, and we should have the results in a couple of days. How would you like us to contact you?"

"Please don't email. I certainly don't want this information in writing anywhere where it might be seen. Call my cell phone. I listed it as my primary contact number," Tanya replied somewhat curtly.

Shortly after the doctor exited the room, a short, middle-aged brunette walked in. "Tanya? I'm Cindy, the phlebotomist for Health Partners. Looks like we need to repeat a blood test for you."

Tanya felt her face turning beet red. "I have to tell you, I'm sure that last test was a mistake. I'm perfectly healthy," she told Cindy.

"This might sting a bit. Please don't move or pull away," Cindy said kindly when she was ready to insert the needle. Once the blood was drawn, Cindy quickly and cautiously disposed of the needle and then sealed the tube of blood inside a plastic bag and placed a bandage on Tanya before removing and disposing of her gloves in a red canister marked "Biohazard."

"Could I feel any more like a leper?," thought Tanya, inwardly cringing from Cindy's defensive body language. "What if I really do have HIV? Is this how people are going to act around me? Will everyone be afraid of me?"

"Okay, you can check out down the hall with the receptionist," Cindy said, dismissing Tanya.

Tanya left the doctor's office, and automatically began walking down the street to her office. She glanced at her watch. "It's four ten. Okay, I have to hold it together for less than an hour before I can head home and figure this out," Tanya thought. And then, her heart sinking, she remembered Seth. "Was that only this morning that I was so excited to accept his dinner invitation? There is absolutely no way that I can go out with him tonight and act normal. I'm going to blow this relationship before it even gets started," she whined to herself. "Of course, if I've got HIV, that's not exactly going to help any relationship to take off," her practical side added.

Back at work, she robotically resumed her tasks, pushing all other thoughts out of her head. At precisely ten after five, Tanya met Seth in the lobby and excused herself from their date, blaming a family crisis that had popped up in the afternoon and agreeing to reschedule dinner for next week.

She maintained her composure until she collapsed onto her couch at home, Shadow thrusting his paws onto her lap and Sir Lance pacing back and forth along the top of the couch behind her head. First silent tears, then heaving sobs racked Tanya as she tried to process the possibility of having HIV disease. "What will my family say? Dad will want to strangle Devon, if not me. What will my friends think? Should I tell anyone at work? Oh my God, what if I gave it to John or Garrett? How will I live with myself? Why didn't I use condoms? Would it have mattered? Should I try to reach Devon? How could I have been so stupid?"

Rapid-fire questions cycled endlessly in her brain, with no answers to be found. At different points, she decided the whole thing was ridiculous and that this angst was for nothing. Then the questions would start again, sending her into a downward spiral. She was numb at work. By the time the phone call came two days later, Tanya felt emotionally drained.

"This is Tanya," she said, her heart pounding as she answered the call from Health Partners.

"Tanya, this is Lori, Dr. Andrews's nurse," said a kind voice. "I'm sorry, but the repeat HIV test is still positive. Dr. Andrews asked me to help you set up an appointment with the infectious disease specialist. I called them, and they can work you in tomorrow morning at ten thirty. Can you make that time?"

Tanya could barely speak. "Um, yes, thank you." She wrote down the office address and phone number, completely in shock.

"Feel free to call us if you have any problems," Lori was saying.

"Sure."

"Tanya, I'm so sorry. It'll be okay. Dr. Fagerberg is the best. She'll take good care of you," Lori said empathetically.

"I'm sorry too," concurred Tanya, ending the call. "Believe me, I'm deeply sorry."

facts

HIV Fact Sheet

What is it?

- HIV stands for human immunodeficiency virus, the virus that causes AIDS (acquired immune deficiency syndrome).

How common is it?

- More than 1.2 million Americans have confirmed HIV infection or AIDS.

- The CDC believes that roughly 14% of infected people in the United States do not know they are infected.

- An estimated 50,000 Americans are newly infected each year, a number that has remained stable in the last several years. There were 47,352 newly diagnosed cases of HIV/AIDS in 2013, 80% male and 20% female.

- According to the CDC, AIDS is 7 times more prevalent in African Americans and 3 times more prevalent in Hispanic Americans than in Caucasian Americans.

How do you get it?

- HIV is transmitted by direct contact between an infected person's blood or body fluids and another person's blood, broken skin, or mucous membranes; therefore, HIV is transmitted by sex (oral, anal, or vaginal) or sharing needles or syringes (which may occur with IV drug use).

- Receptive anal intercourse is the highest-risk type of sex for transmitting HIV (because the lining of the rectum is more fragile than the lining of the vagina).

- In 2015 data analysis confirmed that 25% of new HIV infections were transmitted via heterosexual contact; 63% were transmitted through MSM (men who have sex with men); 8% via injection drug use; and 3% with combined MSM and injection drug use.

- Pregnant women infected with HIV can transmit the virus to their unborn child during pregnancy or delivery. The virus can also be transmitted through breastfeeding.

Where on your body do you get it?

- HIV infects white blood cells, specifically the CD4+T cells. HIV infection itself is not visible on the outside of the body.

How do I know if I have it?

- The only way to know if you have HIV is to be tested, because many people are asymptomatic, on average for up to 10 years after the initial infection. The CDC recommends routine HIV screening for everyone between the ages of 13 and 64 years at least once.

- Some people get a flu-like illness in the first few months of infection. They develop headache, fever, fatigue, and enlarged lymph nodes.

- Blood tests can detect antibodies to HIV, whether or not people have any symptoms. There are three tests: the EIA (enzyme immunoassay), which is a rapid screening test; and the Western blot and the IFA (immunofluorescence assay), which are slower, confirmatory tests. Saliva tests are also available but are less accurate because there are lower levels of antibodies in saliva than in blood.

- Late in the disease, when the immune system is weakened, other symptoms begin to appear, such as frequent yeast infections, unusual rashes, fevers and sweats, weight loss, severe herpes infections, and/or short-term memory loss.

What does it look like?

- While there are some characteristic skin lesions late in the disease, most people with HIV infection look completely normal.

What does it feel like?

- Initially, many people feel tired or have unexplained weight loss, fevers, or chills.

- Lymph nodes may swell and ache (in neck, armpits, or groin).

- Headache, muscle aches, stiff neck, sore throat, fever, and flu-like symptoms may occur in the first few months.

- Many people feel normal and are unaware that they are infected.

How long does it last?

- HIV infections currently last for a lifetime.

Can it be cured?

- Not yet, although treatments are improving every year.

Can HIV be transmitted between homosexual partners?

- Recent data show that 63% of newly HIV-infected individuals in the United States were men who have sex with men.

- There are case reports of woman-to-woman transmission, likely involving menstrual blood or vaginitis, but the rate of transmission is unknown and believed to be very low.

What is AIDS?

- AIDS (acquired immune deficiency syndrome) refers to the most advanced stage of HIV infection. There are set criteria that define it, including blood counts (CD4+T cells < 200) and the presence of at least 1 of 26 infections that wouldn't typically be present in a person with a healthy immune system.

- For untreated HIV disease, the time from initial HIV infection until the development of AIDS can range from a few months to 17 years, with the median time being 10 years. Survival is higher in people who are younger at the time of diagnosis (children or adults under the age of 45).

- CDC data show that 13,712 people in the United States died from AIDS in 2012, and in total to date, approximately 660,000 people in the United States have died from AIDS.

What is the treatment?

- Antiviral medicines called reverse transcriptase inhibitors block the virus from copying itself.

- There are three main classes of drugs, but because HIV can easily become resistant to medicines, HIV disease is usually treated with a combination of drugs, which is more effective.

- Other medicines are added to prevent opportunistic infections (bacterial, viral, and parasitic infections that generally don't make people with normal immune systems ill).

- There can be serious side effects from any of the anti-HIV drugs, so patients must work closely with their doctors to ensure optimal care.

Is there a vaccine?

- Vaccines are undergoing clinical trials but are not available for general use yet.

How about alternative therapies?

- No alternative medicine therapies can cure HIV infection. Vitamin and mineral supplementation is the most prevalent alternative medicine practice among HIV-positive individuals.

- Exercise, including resistance training to build muscle, is encouraged.

- Meditation, yoga, massage, and herbal medicines are also used to complement conventional treatments.

Are there long-term consequences?

- HIV progresses to AIDS, which results in death from opportunistic infections and cancers.

When are you contagious?

- Always.

How do I avoid getting HIV?

- Abstinence from IV drug use and sharing needles and from vaginal, anal, and oral sex will prevent the transmission of HIV.

- Proper and consistent use of condoms decreases transmission of HIV.

- Use fresh condoms with each partner if sharing sex toys or, preferably, do not share sex toys.

- If you are in the healthcare profession, take extra care to avoid contaminated needle sticks (including but not limited to wearing gloves and not recapping needles).

- Limit sexual intimacy to a monogamous relationship in which both parties have tested negative for HIV at least six months after their last sexual contact (or after other high-risk behavior, such as sharing needles).

- PrEP stands for pre-exposure prophylaxis, which means taking medicine before you have high-risk intimacy (such as when you are HIV-negative but your partner in an ongoing relationship has HIV). PrEP is a combination pill of two oral HIV drugs, tenofovir and emtricitabine (brand name: Truvada), and it is taken every day for the prevention of new infection.

If I have HIV, how do I avoid giving it to my partner?

- The only way to be 100% sure not to transmit HIV is to abstain from oral, vaginal, and anal sex and from sharing needles.

- Consistent condom use and PrEP can greatly decrease the transmission of HIV.

Frequently Asked Questions

- **Can you catch HIV from hugging, kissing, or shaking hands with someone who is infected?**
  No. The virus dies when it dries out.

- **Can you catch HIV from a toilet seat?**
  No. HIV dies quickly once it is outside the body.

- **Can you catch HIV from sharing a drinking glass or water fountain?**
  No. The virus can be detected in saliva, but there is no evidence that it can be transmitted by saliva.

- **Can you catch HIV today from a blood transfusion?**
  No. Since 1985, all donated blood in the United States has been tested for HIV antibodies. If you received a blood transfusion prior to 1985, however, you could be at risk.

- **Don't you have to be gay or abuse drugs to catch HIV?**
  No. Data from the CDC show that in the 47,500 cases of newly diagnosed HIV in the United States in 2010 (confirmed in 2015), 63% had male-to-male sexual contact, 8% reported IV drug use, and 3% had male-to-male sexual contact and injection drug use, but 25% had only heterosexual contact and did not use IV drugs. Receptive anal intercourse (in men or women) creates the highest risk for becoming infected with HIV.
  The potential risk assessment is further complicated by the number of men who are on the "down low," meaning they do not consider themselves to be homosexual but do report engaging in male-to-male sexual activities in addition to heterosexual ones.

Additional Information

AIDSinfo
PO Box 4780
Rockville, MD 20849-6303

1-800-HIV-0440 (1-800-448-0440), 1 -888-480-3739 (TTY)
http://aidsinfo.nih.gov

American College of Obstetricians and Gynecologists
PO Box 70620
Washington, DC 20024-9998
1-800-673-8444
www.acog.org/publications/patient_education/bp082.cfm

American Sexual Health Association
PO Box 13827
Research Triangle Park, NC 27709
919-361-8400
www.ashasexualhealth.org/

Centers for Disease Control and Prevention
1600 Clifton Road
Atlanta, GA 30329-4027
1-800-CDC-INFO (1-800-232-4636), 1-888-232-6348 (TTY)
www.cdc.gov/hiv/
HIV Surveillance Report
www.cdc.gov/hiv/library/reports/surveillance/

MedlinePlus
US National Library of Medicine
8600 Rockville Pike
Bethesda, MD 20894
1-888-FIND-NLM (1-888-346-3656) or 301-594-5983
www.nlm.nih.gov/medlineplus/aids.html

HEPATITIS C

17: Shannon

SHANNON RUSHED INTO THE house with her arms full, stumbling over the daily batch of mail. She unloaded the groceries, grabbed snacks for the kids, gathered up the mail, and jumped back into her car, heading to the school to pick up her kids and deliver them to their respective activities. When the last child, Tristan, left the car for his trumpet lesson, she glanced at the mail and noticed an official-looking letter from the blood bank. As Shannon opened the envelope, she privately congratulated herself, thinking that this would likely be a thank you note for her contribution to the church's annual blood drive.

Shannon had been excited to give blood for the first time in her life. The blood bank had just decreased its minimum weight requirement for donors from a hundred and ten pounds to a hundred and five, so Shannon was finally eligible to give the "gift of life." At five foot one (okay, five foot and half an inch, but who's counting?) the former cheerleader and now thirty-eight-year-old PTA president still looked as though she might be a recent college graduate. Strawberry blonde hair, freckles, and dimples completed her cherubic appearance, thanks to her Irish roots. Shannon had such positive energy and enthusiasm that she never lacked for volunteers for any project, no matter how onerous the task. She was the first to jump in and roll up her sleeves to get a job done, and it had always bothered her that she was ineligible to donate blood when she organized the semi-annual blood drive. Shannon smiled as she opened her letter and began to read:

> Dear Mrs. Shannon Mahoney,
>
> Thank you for your recent donation to the Travis County Blood Bank. Unfortunately, we are unable to use your blood, as it tested positive for hepatitis C. Please see your primary care physician for further evaluation.

Shannon's first thought was disappointment. "I finally gave blood, and they couldn't even use it? What a bummer." But as she sat there feeling sorry for herself, her mind began processing the rest of the information. "Now wait a minute," she thought. "Hepatitis C? What on earth is that—some kind of food poisoning? I did have oysters a few weeks ago. Isn't that what causes hepatitis?"

Shannon was puzzled, especially since she hadn't been sick at all. "Oh well," she thought, "maybe it's a mistake. I guess it's time to call our family doctor and get an annual exam." Shannon realized, as she thought about it, that since she had had her tubes tied after the extremely difficult pregnancy with the twins, she had slacked off on getting her yearly physicals. When she was having babies, her gynecologist did her exams. However, since Macy and Mackenzie were born six years ago, Shannon had only made time for one or two physicals. She grabbed her phone, quickly pulled up Dr. Wren's website, and hoped for decent cell service as she called the office.

"Hi. This is Shannon Mahoney, and I'd like to make an appointment with Dr. Wren."

"Okay. Did you have any special concerns, or is this just your routine visit?," inquired the receptionist.

"Well, I am definitely overdue for my annual exam, but I just received a letter from the blood bank saying I've got some kind of hepatitis, so that's why I'm calling now," Shannon replied casually.

"Hepatitis? Oh, that really shouldn't wait until your physical. Dr. Wren is booked for a couple of months for routine annuals. Let's go ahead and make an appointment soon for the hepatitis, and then we'll plug you in for your physical in February, okay?"

"I'm not sick or anything. Can't everything just wait until February?," Shannon inquired as apprehension spawned butterflies in her stomach.

"Actually, no. I'm glad you're feeling well, but I think Dr. Wren would want to see you sooner to discuss your hepatitis. We have an acute care spot open tomorrow morning at ten. Will that work for you?"

Shannon grabbed her day planner and looked at Friday's schedule. "Um, ten will be fine. Is this something I need to be concerned about?," she asked.

"Don't worry. Dr. Wren will answer all your questions at your appointment tomorrow. Please be here fifteen minutes early to fill out paperwork, or you can go online and update them there, and remember to bring your current insurance card. It looks like you've not been in for a while. Are you still on Blue Cross?"

Shannon fumbled through her purse for her insurance card and gave the receptionist all her vital statistics. She was still giving out information when Tristan startled her by jumping into the car and slamming the door as he tossed his trumpet onto the back seat.

"Hey, what's for dinner? I'm starved," he announced.

Shannon finished her phone call and made a reminder for herself for the appointment before she put the car in gear. "How was your lesson?," she asked.

The rest of the evening passed in a blur as she gathered the kids from their activities and managed to get everyone fed, showered, and ready for bed just as her husband, Will, arrived home late from a business meeting.

As they shared a glass of wine together during their nightly ritual of chatting about their day, Shannon mentioned the letter and her doctor's appointment to Will. "So, do you think I got this hepatitis from those oysters we ate last month?," Shannon asked.

"Honestly, honey, I have no idea. I thought hepatitis C was something that drug addicts got," Will said, without thinking.

"Drug addicts? Now how in the world would I get that?," Shannon asked incredulously. "Do you really think it's related to something like that?"

Will shrugged and suggested, "Why not look it up online?"

Shannon reached for her tablet and typed in "hepatitis C." The search engine soon produced more than fourteen million websites. Will looked over her shoulder at the staggering amount of information.

"Why don't you wait and talk with Dr. Wren about it tomorrow?," he asked gently. "You know half those websites are probably totally inaccurate anyway. You're just going to freak yourself out with that stuff. And it sounds like someone is needing you anyway." Will chuckled, as they heard one of the twins calling out "Mom!"

"Just a minute. Let me look at a couple of sites so I can at least ask some intelligent questions tomorrow, okay? Can you check on the kids, and give me some time to read?," Shannon asked.

"Fair enough," Will replied. "I'll be back in ten minutes."

Shannon scanned the search results and clicked on what looked to her to be a reputable site. As she started reading, she realized Will's first instinct had been right. Apparently hepatitis C is a disease that is transmitted through blood—such as by a blood transfusion, IV drug abuse, or sex. To the best of her knowledge, Shannon had never had a blood transfusion. She made a mental note to check her records. Shannon had absolutely never used drugs of any kind, and the only man she had been intimate with was her husband. Since Will had given blood a few times over the years, she assumed he was "clean." "Maybe it was a mistake after all," she thought.

"Shannon, the twins need your help to finish their Brownie project," called Will from the other room. "Can you come here?"

Shannon sighed, but put down the tablet and headed toward the girls' room. She had known that finishing the Brownie "sit-upons" would require some adult help as soon as Macy and Mackenzie had carried them into the minivan. By the time she had the girls tucked away, Shannon was too exhausted to read anymore online.

The next morning was uneventful as Shannon shuttled everyone to school and arrived at Dr. Wren's office. The nurse checked her in, commenting favorably about her weight and low blood pressure.

Shannon handed her the letter from the blood bank to put in her chart.

"Do you think I need to be worried about this?," she asked.

The nurse looked at the sheet and frowned. "Well, hepatitis can be serious, but you certainly look healthy. Let's see what the doctor has to say, okay?"

Dr. Wren came into the room about five minutes later. "Shannon, it's been a while since I've seen you. How are your kids?," she asked with a smile.

"They're all doing well. The twins are big enough to be Brownies already, can you believe it?," Shannon replied. "Anyway, I feel totally fine. Like every mom I know, I have plenty of days where I feel exhausted, but overall, I think I'm pretty healthy. I think I've only been in to see you with a sinus infection or something else minor in the last several years, right? So what's up with this letter? Do you think it's a mistake?" Shannon knew she was rambling a bit, which always happened when she was nervous.

Dr. Wren read the letter. She then started scanning through Shannon's electronic medical record. "It's been quite a while since your last physical, but I don't remember having any special concerns about your liver. Let's see . . ." She stopped and pursed her lips as she reviewed Shannon's old blood test results. "Well, on your last physical three years ago, your labs were completely normal, including your liver functions. Two years before that, you did have a small elevation in your liver enzymes, but we thought that was probably due to your gallstones, remember?"

Shannon nodded. "How could I forget getting my gallbladder removed when Macy and Mackenzie were so young? At least you guys waited 'til after the pregnancy."

Dr. Wren nodded. "Shannon, did you ever have a blood transfusion before you moved here? I know you haven't had one since I've been taking care of you."

"No. Doctors would have told me, right?"

"Absolutely. Now don't be offended, but I need to ask you some more questions, okay?," said the doctor.

Shannon laughed. "I'm a step ahead of you. No, I've never used drugs, and I've only had sex with my husband. Anything else?"

"Is this the first time you've given blood?"

"Yes."

"And did Will give blood this year too?"

"Yes, and he didn't get any letter, if that's where you're headed," replied Shannon.

"And, basically, you've been healthy? No nausea, diarrhea, or unexplained fatigue?," the doctor asked.

"I'm afraid all my fatigue is perfectly explainable." Shannon smiled.

"Let's take a look at you," Dr. Wren said as she reached for her stethoscope. She looked Shannon over head to toe, only pausing for a moment during her exam of Shannon's abdomen. She pointed to Shannon's lower right belly. "Remind me. What's the story behind this?"

Shannon flushed, instinctively reaching to cover her tattoo. "You know, what am I going to say to my kids when they want a tattoo? Now I know why my mom freaked out when I got this shamrock. She kept telling me that I would regret it when I was older. I have to tell you though—it seemed awfully cool when I got it. Right before we graduated, all the cheerleaders wanted to have some permanent reminder of our senior year. Everyone thought we were such 'goody-goodies,' and we kind of wanted to do something rebellious. On our senior spring break trip, we decided to go together and each get a tasteful, small tattoo that would just barely show above our bikinis. Almost all of us went through with it, and I picked a shamrock because I was headed to Notre Dame. At least we decided on a spot that wouldn't be visible with regular clothes on. Who thought back then how it would look after it got stretched out a few times with having kids?"

Dr. Wren smiled. "Well, it's still cute, even if one side got a bit stretched out. My concern is that, apparently, it's your only risk factor for hepatitis C."

Shannon was shocked. "You mean, you can catch it from getting a tattoo? This tattoo is over twenty years old. Wouldn't it have showed up before now?"

Dr. Wren shook her head. "Not necessarily. Do you remember anything about the shop where you got it? I doubt back then that you asked if they sterilized their needles."

"Oh my gosh, I have no idea. We thought it looked like a decent enough place, but it never occurred to any of us that getting a tattoo could be a health risk. Do you really think that's how I got this?"

"Well, assuming that our repeat test today confirms that you really do have hepatitis C, that would be my educated guess. There is some debate in the medical literature about how often it is transmitted that way, but it is a blood-borne disease, so it makes sense to me. Even if they used fresh needles, if they used the same ink for multiple people, it would be contaminated. Having said that, there are many people with hepatitis C who have no obvious risk factors, including tattoos."

"What about my husband, Will? Wouldn't he have it by now if I have had this for over twenty years?," asked Shannon. "And oh my gosh, what about the kids? Could I have given it to them? They've never had any occasion to have their blood drawn." Shannon was starting to panic. Her family was absolutely the most important thing in the world to her, and the thought that she could have harmed them was almost too much for her to tolerate.

Dr. Wren put her hand on Shannon's arm. "Okay, one step at a time. Why don't I let you get dressed, and I'll be right back with some handouts about hepatitis C. It's possible that this was a false positive, but even if you do have it, chances are good that no one else in your family is infected. I promise we'll go over everything, okay?"

By the time Shannon was dressed and feeling more composed, Dr. Wren was back. "Okay, Shannon. The first thing we need to do is to draw your blood today and do another test to confirm whether or not you are truly infected. In the blood-donor population, a positive test can turn out to be wrong up to twenty percent of the time."

"Really?," Shannon asked hopefully.

"Yes. However, let me go ahead and tell you about hepatitis, in case you are truly infected." She handed Shannon an information sheet. "Let's go over this together, okay? First of all, there are different kinds of hepatitis. Hepatitis means inflammation of the liver. It can be infectious, like from hepatitis A, B, or C, or even from another virus such as mono. It can also come from alcoholism or medicines. We worry about hepatitis the most when it becomes chronic, meaning that the inflammation in the liver doesn't go away after the initial illness. With hepatitis C, many people don't remember being ill. The symptoms of early infection can be mild or are often like a case of food poisoning or a stomach virus, with several days of nausea, vomiting, or diarrhea. Then it can be silent for years, not noticed until there is enough inflammation to cause a rise in the blood levels of liver enzymes."

"Like I had with my gallstones?," Shannon interrupted.

"Yes. It is the same enzymes. We'll be checking those today, along with the repeat antibody test for hepatitis C and another test, called "HCV RNA," that checks for the actual virus. We'll also check to see if you have antibodies to hepatitis A and B, and we'll give you immunizations for those if you don't, to avoid any preventable further insult to your liver. Your children are already immunized for hepatitis A and B, by the way. Routine vaccination of kids for hepatitis B began in 1991, and your kids received the hepatitis A vaccine when there was an outbreak in their daycare center. We don't have a shot yet to prevent hepatitis C. If you have had hepatitis C for all these years, your children have a less than five percent chance of having caught it from you when you were pregnant. I know you breastfed them too, and I want to reassure you that hepatitis C is not thought to be transmitted through breast milk."

"Thank goodness for that," said Shannon.

Dr. Wren continued. "What we worry about with hepatitis C is that some people—somewhere between five and twenty percent—go on to develop scarring of the liver, called cirrhosis, and some even go on to develop liver cancer. Hepatitis C is the leading cause for liver transplantation. We do have treatments to prevent the progression of the disease, but there are significant side effects to some treatments. Hopefully, if your hepatitis C antibody is a true positive, the HCV RNA test will be negative, which means your infection has already resolved, so you won't need treatment."

"What else do I need to do? Is there any special diet I need to follow?," asked Shannon.

"Generally, we just want you to maximize your health. Eat right, exercise, and limit alcohol as much as possible. Also, we'll have you avoid acetaminophen, like the brand name Tylenol, as a pain reliever, since it can irritate the liver," replied Dr. Wren.

"So goodbye to wine with dinner."

"At least as a regular event, yes," said Dr. Wren.

"But I'm not contagious if I'm kissing the kids or anything?," Shannon asked.

"Really, it's just spread by blood. You shouldn't share razors or toothbrushes with anyone, but otherwise, it's not that contagious. You don't spread it by general close contact."

"Okay. What about Will? Should we be using condoms? That would certainly be ironic after being married this long and having my tubes tied," Shannon said.

"In your situation, I wouldn't necessarily recommend that. As you've said, he's potentially been exposed for over two decades. Studies show that in long-term monogamous couples in which only one person is positive for hepatitis C, the transmission rate is less than one percent per year."

"But we should test him and the kids?"

Dr. Wren smiled. "If today's test confirms the blood bank's test, then yes, we will test them all, but remember, the chances of Will and the children being infected are very low. We should have your results early next week, and we'll contact you as soon as we have them. Any other questions?"

"I guess not. I hope this shamrock has some Irish luck left in it," Shannon said.

The phone call came Tuesday morning. Dr. Wren's nurse was pleasant enough, but the information was not. The second tests confirmed hepatitis C, including showing that the virus was still present. The doctor wanted her to make a follow-up appointment to discuss the results. Shannon hung up the phone, somewhat in shock. "All of this, from a tattoo?," she thought. "Maybe moms *are* always right."

18: Luke

LUKE PUSHED BACK FROM his desk, swiveling in his soft leather chair to better absorb the spectacular view from his home office's picture window. Mount Crested Butte's sheer cliffs were beginning to cast shadows from the setting sun. Looking closely, Luke could make out the proud profile of a Native American's face along the far southern edge, where the rocky landslides met the aspens. The cool weather and shorter days were coaxing the aspens to become golden yellow, glistening between the evergreens.

"I can't believe I'm finally free to spend a whole month in the fall up here," Luke gloated. Luke was the president of his own startup software company. As long as he had good Internet access, he was free to travel away from his native San Jose, California. Throughout his twenties and early thirties, Luke had hopped flights to Crested Butte any time he could put together a three-day weekend. In the summers, he learned to whitewater raft and kayak. In the springs, Luke hit the single-track in this birthplace of mountain biking. For the two weeks of the fall color change, though, it was all about hiking. From Green Lake Trail to West Maroon Pass, Luke explored every open trail, inhaling the crisp scents and perfecting digital photographs of the aspens as they evolved.

When his company went public, Luke made millions of dollars. That had happened about a year ago, and his only major splurge was this new home in Crested Butte. Located on the back nine of the golf course, it gave him a view of the town from one side of his house and this amazing view of the mountain from the other. The home was finished with high-end amenities, from a drop-down big-screen television to a climate-controlled wine cellar. "Life simply doesn't get any better than this," Luke said to his faithful companion, Stash, a three-year-old Labrador mix, who wagged his tail enthusiastically in agreement.

"Ellen would be awfully jealous of our wine collection, although she wouldn't fully appreciate the town," mused Luke. Ellen was Luke's last girlfriend. Their brief but intense six-month relationship had been a fun diversion, but Luke didn't particularly miss her. Ellen had originally been his accountant. Shortly after Luke's company went public, Ellen had blindsided Luke by showing up unannounced at his condo with a bottle of wine to celebrate his newfound success. Unfortunately, it turned out that their only common interest was the profits from his company. Ellen enjoyed museums, fine dining, and shopping. Luke favored outdoor recreation, pizza, and beer. Luke gained an appreciation for excellent wine during the brief relationship but had also realized he preferred the easygoing companionship of a dog over complex human interactions.

Luke refocused on the task at hand. "Let me get through my email, and we'll head out for a hike. Okay, Stash?" He turned back to the desk and started answering and deleting emails methodically. "Stanford wants money again," he said. "But not today!" He laughed, deleting his alma mater's request. "Looks like this is my new life insurance approval, Stash. Maybe I'll make you my beneficiary." Luke chuckled at the dog.

"Wait, what's this?" Luke grimaced as he read through the email. "Apparently, they don't like my liver. I need to have further tests and clearance from my regular doctor. I bet I can get in to see Dr. Hunter this week. Of course, we know what she's going to say, don't we, buddy?" Luke scratched his dog behind the ears. Stash licked Luke's hand and barked. "That's right, Stash. She's going to tell me to stop drinking. Oh well, I'll call for an appointment tomorrow."

Luke had seen a local doctor, Dr. Hunter, for a variety of minor ailments and injuries over the years. She had treated a broken arm from snowboarding, road rash from mountain-bike crashes, and a few episodes of alcohol-related gastritis. He walked out of the study without another thought regarding his health and grabbed the leash. "Come on, let's go hike the upper loop."

A couple of days later, Luke had his appointment with Dr. Hunter to get her opinion on the abnormal liver tests. After examining him, the doctor sat across from Luke, flipping through the back of his chart and comparing the new numbers to the earlier lab results.

"Really, Dr. Hunter, you should be using electronic medical records by now," Luke teased.

"Not in a tiny private practice in the mountains, Luke." She laughed. "I can't afford it, and even if I could, frankly I like the old charts. They don't stop working when the power goes out."

"Fair enough," replied Luke, "but I bet it would make things easier."

Dr. Hunter shrugged as she continued flipping pages. "Luke, looking back over the sporadic labs we have on you for the last seven or eight years, I only see one other time when your liver functions were abnormal. Three years ago, when you came in with stomach pain, your enzymes were elevated, but it looks like the tests were never repeated as I had suggested. Knowing you, you went back to California and forgot about it," she chastised.

"Well, I'm here for a whole month this time, so you should be able to fix me up," he countered.

"We'll see. Let's go over a few things. Are you having nausea, vomiting, diarrhea, or pain?," she asked.

"Not at all," Luke reassured her.

"How about your reflux? Are you having any heartburn?," asked the doctor.

"You know, it comes and goes, but it hasn't been bad recently," admitted Luke. "I've been taking some antacids but no prescription medicines, like before."

"And you're not taking any medicines on a regular basis, including over-the-counter stuff like Tylenol, right?," she asked.

"No, I don't like pills, so I rarely even take an aspirin," Luke answered.

"How much alcohol are you drinking these days?," the doctor inquired.

"More than you'd approve of," said Luke with a grin.

"Seriously, how many drinks per week?"

"During the week, most days I'll have a beer or a couple of glasses of wine with dinner, but I'll admit that on the weekends, I may have more in a night if I'm out listening to music."

"And how's your caffeine intake? Still measuring by the pot?," asked Dr. Hunter.

"I switched to decaf for a while, but yes, I'm back to fully leaded coffee, a couple of pots per day."

"Well, at least you don't smoke or dip tobacco," said the doctor.

"But between your caffeine and alcohol, I'm not surprised you're still having reflux symptoms. It sounds like alcohol is the most likely cause for your abnormal liver tests. Since there is nothing else abnormal in your physical exam or the rest of your bloodwork, let's have you abstain from alcohol for about ten days, and then we'll repeat your lab work. Enjoy the fall colors," she added, handing Luke his lab slip, "and I'll see you late next week."

The time passed quickly for Luke. During the days, he enjoyed exploring new hikes with Stash, watching the dog scout for deer and small mammals as he followed his keen nose off the trails. The late afternoons and evenings were tied up with work on the computer and slugging down mugs of special blends from his favorite local coffee shop, Camp 4 Coffee. Although he found it a bit difficult to wind down at the end of the night without his evening drink, the natural discipline that had carried him to corporate success kicked in, and Luke strictly followed the doctor's advice.

Back in the doctor's office, Luke and Dr. Hunter were both disappointed by his blood test results. "Your liver functions are still significantly elevated, Luke, so now we need to start looking for other causes," she said.

"You sound so serious. How bad can it be, with everything else being normal?," asked Luke.

Dr. Hunter was pragmatic. "First, we'll test your blood for the different types of infectious hepatitis. I know you've had the hepatitis B series of shots, but we'll make sure your antibodies show immunity, plus we'll check for hepatitis C and A. Type A is unlikely, since your enzymes have been abnormal for a couple of years, and type A doesn't go on to cause long-term problems."

"Were the hepatitis B shots the ones I got before traveling to China a few years ago?"

"Yes, by my notes in your chart, it looks like you received those in California around four years ago."

"Are those vaccines very effective?," he asked.

"Absolutely. Hepatitis B is an enormous global health problem. More than two billion people worldwide have been infected, and of that group, more than three hundred and fifty million people have become chronic carriers of the infection. Complications of the infection account for over a million deaths annually. The hepatitis B vaccine is ninety-five percent effective in preventing chronic infections from developing. Here in the United States, there are more than a million carriers of hepatitis B, but since we began recommending the universal vaccination of children in 1991, the overall rate of acute cases of hepatitis B has dropped nearly seventy percent, and almost ninety percent in children and adolescents."

"That's impressive. So hopefully, for me, this means that I shouldn't have hepatitis B. Is there anything else you need to test?," asked Luke.

"We'll also check for HIV, although according to your history you are low risk, with no drug use, no prior STIs, and only a few sexual partners," Dr. Hunter said, referring to notes in the chart. "Unless there's been any change in that lately?"

"Hardly," Luke replied. "Truthfully, relationships take too much time. I've always been kind of an introvert, and in general, I'm happier by myself or hanging out with my Stash."

"Referring to your dog, not drugs, right?" Dr. Hunter laughed. "Because that would definitely change your risk factors."

"Absolutely," confirmed Luke.

"Anyway, since you have a completely normal white blood cell count and no physical complaints, it's unlikely to be a mono syndrome, which is something else that can cause transient liver function abnormalities."

"Are there any other tests besides bloodwork?," he asked.

"If these tests all come back normal, then we'll have you get an abdominal ultrasound."

"What's that for?," asked Luke.

"It would provide a good look at your liver and your gallbladder. Sometimes, gallstone disease will cause liver function abnormalities, even without symptoms. Let's take it one step at a time though, Luke. We'll get your extra blood tests back in a few days, and we'll go from there, okay?"

"All right," agreed Luke. "You know, maybe it's my caffeine. I'll switch to decaf and see if that makes any difference while we're waiting on the other results."

"It certainly won't hurt, Luke, except possibly for the withdrawal headache," she smiled wryly.

The next Monday, Luke was back in the exam room again. Dr. Hunter came in and sat down with a concerned look on her face.

"Luke, it looks like we've got an answer to why your liver enzymes are abnormal. Your hepatitis C blood test results came back positive."

"Meaning that I've got hepatitis C?," echoed Luke skeptically.

"Yes, I'm afraid so."

"Seriously? I thought only drug addicts got that," exclaimed Luke.

"Well, people who use IV drugs certainly are at high risk for it, but up to twenty percent of people with hepatitis C have no identifiable risk factor except intercourse."

"Sex, huh?"

Dr. Hunter continued. "On the plus side, your tests show that your body has immunity to types A and B, so we don't need to worry about getting you up to speed on those shots."

"Why does that matter?," asked Luke.

"If a person develops one type of hepatitis, we immunize them against the other types to minimize any potential further damage to the liver," explained Dr. Hunter.

"Makes sense," Luke agreed.

Dr. Hunter looked back at the lab results. "Another bit of good news is that your HIV test was negative."

"I'd hope so," Luke remarked flippantly. "So, cut to the chase. What does this mean? Can you treat me?"

Dr. Hunter shook her head. "No. I'm going to refer you to a gastrointestinal specialist in Colorado Springs. Dr. Swegler specializes in liver diseases, especially hepatitis C. You may not even need any treatment now, but I'd like you to get established with someone in Colorado if you're going to be up here more consistently. Either that or you can see someone back in California. We're too small locally to have this kind of specialist here."

"What will he do for me?," asked Luke.

"*She* will do some additional tests to decide if you meet the criteria for treatment, possibly including a liver biopsy," replied Dr. Hunter.

"That doesn't sound too fun," commented Luke. "Can't you tell how bad the disease is by my liver enzymes?"

"No. The enzyme levels actually do not correlate well with how severe the hepatitis C infection is," said the doctor.

"Even though they went back to normal for a while, before they went up again? It seems to me that should be a good sign," rationalized Luke.

"That would sound logical, but with hepatitis C, the blood enzyme levels can fluctuate up and down regardless of the disease progression."

"Is this a really bad disease? What's it going to do to me?"

"Well, like any chronic disease, there is a whole spectrum of how hepatitis C can appear," explained Dr. Hunter. "More than three million Americans have chronic hepatitis C, with roughly thirty thousand new cases identified each year. Up to eighty percent of those people have no symptoms at all. Surprisingly, fifteen to thirty percent of people infected with hepatitis C will spontaneously clear the virus and any liver damage within six months, for reasons unknown at this time. The other seventy to eighty-five percent will have persistent infection. If symptoms are present, they are usually vague, manifesting as fatigue, decreased appetite, muscle or joint aches, or abdominal discomfort."

The doctor continued. "I assume you'll want to know the end point, Luke, so let me tell you that, typically, the disease takes up to twenty or thirty years to cause serious liver damage, with scarring called cirrhosis occurring in ten to twenty percent of chronic carriers. Drinking alcohol is the number one aggravating factor that accelerates this disease. Only one in twenty people who become chronic carriers will develop liver cancer, but liver cancer has a very high mortality rate. As a result, hepatitis C is the leading reason for liver transplantation in the United States."

Luke processed what Dr. Hunter had explained, and then in his typical get-to-work attitude asked, "So what do we need to do now? Is there anything urgent?"

"Really, I'd simply advise you to avoid anything that is tough on the liver, so no products that contain acetaminophen, like Tylenol, and I'd recommend no alcohol."

"None, or moderation?," asked Luke hopefully.

"None. You've already got this hepatitis virus insulting your liver, so you want to avoid anything that will potentially further irritate it. When all's said and done, you basically want to do everything you can to maximize good health. That includes exercise, diet, and a positive attitude."

"Well, I'm positive I'll miss my wine," quipped Luke. "What else do I need to know about this? Is the only way to get it through sex?"

"Hepatitis C is transmitted by blood or body fluids. I know you don't do IV drugs, and you haven't had a blood transfusion, so presumably you caught this through sex. You can also get it by sharing razors or toothbrushes with someone who is infected, but it's still more likely from intercourse. Also, it's possible to get hepatitis C from tattoos, but unless I missed it, you don't have one, do you?," asked the doctor.

"No way. I can't stand needles," shuddered Luke.

"Obviously, you should let any prior partners know, so they can get tested too," said Dr. Hunter.

"That'll be a great email, won't it?," said Luke sarcastically. "Hi there. We haven't spoken in nearly ten years, but I simply wanted to say thanks for the disease you gave me."

"And any future partners," Dr. Hunter continued, choosing to ignore his remark. "Also, you shouldn't donate blood, semen, or organs."

"Again, the needle phobia," Luke reminded the doctor. "I never have donated blood, though I've always felt guilty about that, and I hope I'm not headed for organ donation any time soon."

"I'm just trying to be thorough," chastised Dr. Hunter. "You never know when a cousin might need a kidney or something."

"As long as you didn't mean organ donation after my imminent death," responded Luke.

"Absolutely not. Seriously, Luke, people with hepatitis C can remain asymptomatic for decades, and our treatments are getting better all the time. With your needle phobia, though, I do think I ought to tell you that one of the antiviral treatments, interferon, is actually in shot form."

"Great. And what about that liver biopsy that you mentioned earlier? I'm assuming that involves a big needle." Luke tried to joke.

"That one is long, but skinny," smiled the doctor. "Seriously, though, let's not get ahead of ourselves. You may not even need a liver biopsy at this point. There is some controversy over the timing of liver biopsies in patients with hepatitis C. Your liver enzymes are moderately elevated, but you have no other bloodwork abnormalities, and you don't have any physical findings that suggest advancing liver disease. It will be up to your liver specialist to determine whether or not they would recommend a biopsy at this point. I will tell you it is very individualized treatment, depending on both patient and doctor preferences."

"So the doctor in Colorado might have a different opinion than one back in California?," asked Luke.

"Exactly. If I were you, I'd choose a gastrointestinal specialist in the state where you plan to spend the majority of your time for the next several years," suggested Dr. Hunter.

"For right now, I'd have to choose California, I guess," answered Luke. "Partly because I don't want to waste any time I've got up here trekking several hours over to Colorado Springs, but mainly because I need to be back in San Jose for probably six or seven months out of the next twelve."

"Let me know if you change your mind, and our office will get you Dr. Swegler's information over in the Springs," offered the doctor. "Do you have any other questions?"

"I hate to ask, but this whole thing came about because my new life insurance carrier found those high liver enzymes. They said that I would need clearance from my regular physician. I suppose we have to tell them that I've been diagnosed with hepatitis C, right?," asked Luke.

"Ethically, yes, that is the correct answer. You might want to wait until you see the liver specialist though, so he or she can better assess your prognosis. I'd imagine that a life insurance company would not be too thrilled about this diagnosis, the same as they are not happy about any chronic disease. Every company is different, however, so I can't tell you how they will react specifically. I would assume this diagnosis may be grounds either to deny you coverage or to simply raise your rates," said Dr. Hunter.

"I'll be looking into it. Can I get a copy of all my labs from this month to take with me back to California?"

"Yes. I'll have the folks in the front get you a full set. Best of luck, Luke," said Dr. Hunter, standing up and shaking his hand.

"Thanks. It sounds like I'll need it," responded Luke.

Back at home, Luke sat down in front of his computer, much to the disappointment of Stash, who pawed at Luke's leg for attention, hoping for a walk. Luke rubbed Stash's head halfheartedly but focused his attention on his email address book. "I wonder if this email is even current," he mused as he clicked on the address of an old girlfriend. "She'll be surprised to hear from me outside of the holidays."

Brenda was Luke's last serious relationship, but she seemed to harbor no ill will toward Luke, staying in touch through an annual exchange of Christmas cards. While he typically sent cards with offbeat holiday humor, Brenda's cards were classic family portraits, frequently involving Santa hats. She had become a university professor in biochemistry and was happily married to another PhD. Luke hoped she did not have this same diagnosis. He typed "old friend" into the subject box and tabbed down to construct the email.

"Dear Brenda," he began. "What do I say?," thought Luke, rarely at a loss for words. His blunt, less-than-polished conversational style had never been his greatest asset. Luckily for him, his computer engineering skills and creative mathematical mind were the primary necessary tools for success in his world.

Luke moved the mouse and clicked back on the subject box, deleting "old friend" and entering "hepatitis C." He jumped back down to the text and kept it brief.

> Dear Brenda,
> I'm feeling completely normal but have just been diagnosed with hepatitis C during some bloodwork for an insurance physical. My doctor suggested that I let any previous sexual partners know, so they can get screened too. No clue where I got this or how long I've had it. I hope it wasn't from you.
> Let me know,
> Luke

Luke reread his note, and though the last couple of lines didn't quite sound right, he clicked "send" before editing anything. The other two women he had slept with would be more challenging to locate.

Skye Smith was a girl that Luke had an off-and-on relationship with over several years. Luke had heard through the grapevine a few years back that Skye was doing some kind of volunteer work in Africa. Between her common last name and her global travels, Luke was doubtful of reaching her. He did a few web searches but only discovered links that were no longer current. That one would have to wait.

Finally, there was Ellen, the accountant. From his understanding of the timing of hepatitis C, it seemed more likely that he might have exposed Ellen than vice versa. Luke considered calling her but really didn't want the hassle. He settled instead for another succinct email. Under subject, he again listed "hepatitis C." Scrolling down, he typed:

> Ellen,
> Recent bloodwork showed I have hepatitis C. Doctors recommend that all my previous partners be tested.

But how should he sign it? "Sorry"? "Good luck"? "Sincerely"? Nothing seemed appropriate. Luke remembered how Ellen used to say that she loved the diversion from her world of finance when her computer announced, "You've got mail."

"This email certainly won't bring a smile to her face. How will she react when she sees it?," Luke wondered. "At least I had it broken to me in stages." However, Luke's pragmatic mind kicked in at that point: "Well, it's the information that's important, not the acknowledgment." He merely added his name without any closing salutation. "After seeing the word 'hepatitis,' Ellen won't care about the rest, no matter what I say," he concluded, and with that thought he clicked "send."

He leaned back, pushing away from his computer and stretching his arms. Stash jumped up, interpreting Luke's movements as a sign that it was time to head outside. He wagged his tail and looked up expectantly. Luke had originally intended to start work on some business proposals after he dashed off his personal emails, but distracted by Stash's reaction, he changed his plan.

"This hepatitis C mess is a lot to process, Stash. I think you've got the right idea. There's no point in trying to work right now." Luke stood and grabbed the dog's leash. "Come on, let's go for a hike. The fresh air will do us both some good. I am not going to let this diagnosis rule my life. Dr. Hunter said that I need to maximize my health, and I can't think of a better place to accomplish that than right here in these beautiful mountains. One challenge at a time, we'll conquer this. Let's go."

facts

Hepatitis C (HCV) Fact Sheet

What is it?

- Hepatitis C is an RNA virus, part of the hepatitis family, which includes hepatitis types A, B, C, D, and E.

How common is it?

- The CDC estimates that between 2.7 million and 3.9 million Americans (1.3% of the population) and 170 million people worldwide are infected with HCV.

- In 2012, there were an estimated 21,870 acute cases of hepatitis C.

How do you get it?

- Infected blood or body fluids transmit infection through transfusions, shared needles, or sexual intercourse, or from mother to fetus.

- Since 1992, screening for HCV has caused transfusion-related cases of HCV to drop to less than 1 per million units of blood.

- Sexual transmission of hepatitis C is thought to be inefficient, but the actual percentage of any type of sexual transmission for hepatitis C is unknown. Up to 20% of people with hepatitis C have no known risk factor beyond intercourse.

Where on your body do you get it?

- HCV primarily affects the liver.

How do I know if I have it?

- 60%–70% of people infected with HCV are asymptomatic.

- Blood tests check for antibodies to hepatitis A, B, and C.

- Hepatitis C is often a slowly progressive disease; it can be 10–40 years until serious liver damage occurs.

- 1 in 10 people with HCV have no identifiable risk factors.

What does it look like?

- Usually there are no obvious visible signs of HCV infection.

- Jaundice—yellow eyes and skin—occurs in 20%–30% of people with HCV.

What does it feel like?

- Many people feel completely normal.
- Nonspecific complaints of fatigue, nausea, loss of appetite, or abdominal pain occur in 10%–20% of people with HCV.
- Headache, muscle aches, stiff neck, sore throat, fever, and flu-like symptoms can occur.

How long does it last?

- The incubation period, the time from exposure until the virus is detectable by laboratory testing, is 2–26 weeks.
- 75%–85% of infections become chronic.
- Of chronic infections, 20% lead to cirrhosis (scarring of the liver).
- Of those with cirrhosis, 25% progress to liver failure.
- Once cirrhosis develops, the risk of getting hepatocellular (liver) cancer is 1%–4% per year.
- Roughly 10,000 people die per year in the United States from complications of HCV.

Can it be cured?

- Not yet, although lasting clearance (meaning no detectable virus) can occur in 10%–40% of infected patients treated with interferon and ribavirin. Relapse, however, is not uncommon.
- Reinfection in transplanted livers is common.

What is the treatment?

- New interferon-free, oral medications have simplified treatment for the majority of patients diagnosed with hepatitis C.

- Other treatments that include injectable interferon in combination with ribavirin or other antiviral drugs have a higher incidence of serious side effects, including depression, flu-like symptoms, nausea, headaches, and blood abnormalities.

How about alternative therapies?

- Stress reduction, a healthy diet, and abstaining from alcohol help to improve overall health in patients with chronic hepatitis.

Are there long-term consequences?

- End-stage liver disease from HCV is the cause of over half of the liver transplants performed in the United States each year.

- 80% of HCV infections become chronic.

When are you contagious?

- Always, but not through casual contact—only by sharing infected blood or body fluids.

Can hepatitis C be transmitted between homosexual partners?

- Yes. Exact transmission rates between homosexual partners, however, are unknown.

How do I avoid getting hepatitis C?

- Do not share needles.

- Do not share razors or toothbrushes.

- Do not use shared body-piercing equipment or tattoo needles or ink.
- Abstain from sexual intercourse with partners with hepatitis C or with unknown hepatitis C status.

If I have hepatitis C, how do I avoid giving it to my partner?

- Do not share needles, razors, toothbrushes, or body-piercing equipment.
- Condoms decrease the transmission of hepatitis C.

Frequently Asked Questions

➤ **Does one hepatitis vaccine prevent all types?**
No. The hepatitis A vaccine prevents only type A, and the hepatitis B vaccine only prevents type B. There is no vaccine for type C.

➤ **Can you get hepatitis C from kissing?**
No. HCV is not spread from kissing or casual contact.

➤ **Can you catch HCV from sharing razors?**
Yes. Razors, IV needles, acupuncture needles, tattoo needles, toothbrushes, and body-piercing equipment that have been used on a person with HCV can transmit the virus to another person.

➤ **If you are in a monogamous relationship with someone who has HCV, what is the chance you will catch it?**
Less than 1% per year, and less than 3% long term, assuming you have no other risk factors.
Other coexisting STIs, particularly HIV disease, increase the risk of transmission significantly.
Higher-risk sexual practices, such as intercourse during menses or sexual activity that produces mucosal trauma, can also increase transmission.

➤ **If a healthcare worker is stuck with a needle exposed to HCV, what is their chance of developing HCV infection?** Approximately 2%.

Additional Information

American Liver Foundation
39 Broadway, Suite 2700
New York, NY 10006
212-668-1000
www.liverfoundation.org/

Centers for Disease Control and Prevention
1600 Clifton Road
Atlanta, GA 30329-4027
1-800-CDC-INFO (1-800-232-4636), 1-888-232-6348 (TTY)
www.cdc.gov/ncidod/diseases/hepatitis/c/

HCV Advocate
PO Box 15144
Sacramento, CA 95813
www.hcvadvocate.org/

Hepatitis Foundation International
8121 Georgia Avenue, Suite 350
Silver Spring, MD 20910
1-800-891-0707
www.hepfi.org/

MedlinePlus
US National Library of Medicine
8600 Rockville Pike
Bethesda, MD 20894
1-888-FIND-NLM (1-888-346-3656) or 301-594-5983
www.nlm.nih.gov/medlineplus/hepatitisc.html

Thuluvath, Paul J. *Hepatitis C: A Complete Guide for Patients and Families*. Baltimore, MD: Johns Hopkins University Press, 2015.

SYPHILIS

19: Gavin

GAVIN SEARCHED THROUGH THE magazines in the doctor's office lobby, pleasantly surprised to see a current issue of *People*. "Where is it?," he wondered, flipping quickly past the articles and lingering briefly over the advertisements. "Ah, yes, there I am." He smiled smugly to himself. "Look at those abs. Nice six-pack, if I do say so myself. Arms could use a little work though." As Gavin compared his biceps to the photo, he was dismayed once again at the red bumps covering his forearms and palms. "I sure hope we get an answer this time," he thought.

Gavin depended on his physical appearance for his paycheck. Though he had been a model for years, Gavin was trying to break into the acting business. His agent was fairly confident that Gavin would get a second callback from his latest audition but had warned Gavin that his rash had better be gone by then, or he would lose the part.

About two weeks ago, Gavin had begun to notice small red circles on his palms after using a new moisturizing lotion. The circles became bumps and quickly spread up his forearms. Gavin had gone to a clinic, where he was given a steroid cream and told to stop using the new body lotion. Unfortunately, the rash seemed to worsen in the next week. When Gavin called the clinic for further advice, they referred him to Dr. Coleman, a dermatologist.

Gavin had been slightly offended by her initially. In contrast to his encounter at the clinic, Dr. Coleman had put on gloves before examining his rash and had proceeded to ask him rather embarrassing questions.

"Gavin, have you ever had any sexually transmitted infections, and if so, which ones?," Dr. Coleman had inquired.

"Well, yes," Gavin had answered, though he didn't see the relevance to the red bumps on his arms. "I was treated for gonorrhea once and chlamydia a couple of times over the years. But never herpes," he had added defensively.

"What about HIV or syphilis?," she had asked.

"No. I was last tested for HIV around a year ago, and it was negative," he had replied proudly.

During that visit, Dr. Coleman took a small biopsy from his wrist area, assuring Gavin that the scar would be minimal. She also ordered his blood drawn and asked Gavin to come in for the results in three days.

So here he sat, absentmindedly rubbing his arms, as was his recent habit, waiting to get some answers.

"Gavin?," called the attractive blonde medical assistant from the doorway.

Gavin recognized her from his previous visit. "That's me, and you're Amanda, right?" He flashed a winning smile in her direction and casually put the magazine on the end table, still folded open to his ad.

Amanda coolly directed Gavin into an exam room, not responding to his usually successful flirtatiousness. Instead, she simply indicated he should sit in the chair, dryly noting, "Dr. Coleman will be in momentarily."

"Maybe I'm losing my touch," Gavin mused. Amanda had seemed interested in him earlier in the week but was clearly giving him the cold shoulder today. "Nah, she must be having a bad day," he decided.

Dr. Coleman entered shortly after Amanda left and cut right to the chase as she sat down in front of Gavin. "Well, my suspicions were correct. Gavin, you have syphilis, secondary syphilis, to be exact."

"On my hands?" Gavin recoiled. "Don't you get that on your, uh, privates?"

"Yes, that is typically the location of the initial lesion," said the doctor.

"But I haven't had any red bumps down there, and believe me, I would know," said Gavin defensively.

"Actually, you'd be surprised how often people don't know they have STIs," responded Dr. Coleman. "In the case of syphilis, the initial lesion is usually a single, painless ulcer that shows up anywhere from nine to thirty days after exposure and lasts from three to six weeks. It's most often on the penis in men, but it could have been in your mouth, where you might not have noticed it. Have you had any new sexual partners in the last few months?"

"Plenty, but no one gets syphilis anymore," protested Gavin.

"I'll grant you that it's the least common sexually transmitted infection in the United States, but there are still over fifty-five thousand new syphilis cases reported every year," said Dr. Coleman.

"So I got lucky?" Gavin tried to joke.

"Frankly, yes. The majority of the cases of syphilis that I see now are in my patients who have HIV disease, but your HIV test came back negative. Syphilis we can cure, HIV we cannot," responded Dr. Coleman matter-of-factly.

"Thank goodness for small favors," Gavin smirked. "So what's the cure?"

"Plain, old-fashioned penicillin," answered Dr. Coleman.

"So what about this rash? I still don't get how a rash on my arms is from syphilis."

"Well, the first lesion of syphilis is that painless ulcer I mentioned, and even if it is untreated, that initial spot will heal. But if proper antibiotics are not taken, syphilis then emerges as what you've got, secondary syphilis, which is typically non-itchy red marks and bumps on the skin, especially on the palms or soles of the feet. That was the clue for me to check for syphilis, by the way. Not too many rashes involve the palms. The timing with your new body lotion threw off your first examiner, but I had the benefit of seeing that steroids didn't help and was able to think a little broader," she said modestly.

"And what would have happened if I didn't come in now?," Gavin asked.

"The rash would have eventually disappeared, but it often recurs," explained the doctor. "The worst part is that you can develop tertiary syphilis, which can enter your brain and other organs, causing mental illness, deafness, blindness, and/or death. They call syphilis the great imitator, because when it gets to that stage, it can look like many other diseases."

"Then I guess I am lucky that I came in," said Gavin. "So you're telling me that penicillin will make my rash go away and never come back, and I won't develop any of these worse signs of syphilis?"

"That's correct. Well, as long as . . ." Dr. Coleman paused.

"As long as what?"

"As long as you don't get reinfected," replied the doctor. "Having syphilis once does not protect you from getting it again. It sounds like you're unsure where you caught it, so if you have unprotected sex of any type, you can catch it again. Please advise any sexual partners you've had in the last several months that they must get tested and treated to stop the spread of this disease. Also, since you have secondary syphilis, you need to know that those red bumps are teeming with the bacteria that cause syphilis, so there is the possibility that you infected people who touched them."

"Including the people at the first clinic?," Gavin asked with surprise.

"In theory, anyone who touched your rash without wearing gloves, especially if they had any breaks in their skin," confirmed Dr. Coleman.

"Actually, they may be the only ones," said Gavin. "I've been so self-conscious about this rash that I've been covering it up most of the time."

"They do need to be told. Then, I suggest you go back to your regular doctor, to be tested for all of the sexually transmitted infections as well as for follow-up blood tests for both HIV and syphilis.

I'd also suggest that you refrain from unprotected intimacy in the future." Dr. Coleman finished, "Amanda will be back in with your penicillin shot and a handout on syphilis and other STIs."

Gavin chuckled at the thought of Amanda returning. "No wonder she was aloof today. Really, though, what's the big deal? As they say, I've got nothing penicillin won't cure, and once this rash is gone, who wouldn't want a piece of this?," he arrogantly concluded.

Amanda, for her part, could no longer see the handsome stud she had flirted with earlier in the week. When she administered the penicillin shot, all Amanda saw was a conceited model who had clearly slept with at least one person too many.

20: Liz

"Thank you, everyone, and good night. Look for us next week at Club Heat!," Liz croaked into the microphone over the exuberant crowd. To herself, she added, "Yeah, Club Heat, where I'll be puking in between sets if this so-called morning sickness doesn't let up."

"Great jamming on that last song, Lizzy," congratulated Zane, her boyfriend and the lead guitarist in their band.

"Yeah, you should be pregnant more often," joked the drummer, Jared. "I think it makes your voice sexy, and everyone's definitely loving your new cleavage."

Liz rolled her eyes at Jared, retorting, "My voice is husky from throwing up, and before you know it, my belly will be bigger than my breasts, so enjoy them while you can. Pregnancy is not so great from my end."

"Hey, Liz, be careful what you say. That's my little rock star you've got cooking in there," teased Zane.

"Well, *our* little rock star better start letting me get some rest," Liz answered. Glancing at her watch, she added, "Speaking of rest, are you coming with me to my doctor's appointment in six hours?"

Zane groaned. "What were you thinking, getting an eight o'clock appointment when we had a late gig the night before?"

"My thinking was that this's the time they asked me to come in when they called a few days ago, and since they're squeezing me in, I can't be choosy," snapped Liz.

"Fine, I'll go. Do we get to see the little rocker this time?," Zane asked.

"I have no idea, but I'll bet we'll at least hear his heartbeat again," said Liz, packing away her guitar and handing the case to Zane. "Thanks for carrying my other baby."

"Anything for you, babe." Zane smiled.

Only a few hours later, Liz was sitting in the obstetrician's exam room waiting for the doctor. She had decided to let Zane sleep in, knowing that he had to be at his day job at noon and really needed the rest. Liz was snoozing on the exam table when the doctor finally arrived.

"Sorry for the wait. I had an emergency delivery," Dr. Garcia apologized as she entered.

"No problem, I got a little nap," said Liz.

"Is the morning sickness easing up yet?," asked the doctor.

"Actually, it's minimal in the mornings, but afternoons and nights are pretty tough," admitted Liz.

"Well, hang in there. You're almost past the first trimester, so it should get better soon," said Dr. Garcia. "Now, we called you back in because there was a problem on your initial blood tests, Liz. Unfortunately, you have syphilis."

Liz laughed. "Yeah, right."

"It's not a laughing matter, Liz. I'm serious," chastised the doctor.

Liz sat up straight. "Are you for real? How can I have syphilis and not know it?"

"It's pretty common for people to be unaware of syphilis. That's one reason it's a required test for all pregnant women. Luckily, the rest of your screening tests—HIV, hepatitis C, gonorrhea, and chlamydia—were all negative. The first sign of syphilis is a sore in the vagina, anus, or mouth, but it's painless and goes away on its own, so many people are unaware of it. Although the ulcer goes away, the infection persists, however, and the second stage of syphilis is a rash that can come and go for weeks, usually on the hands," explained Dr. Garcia.

"Oh man, I had a rash on my palms all last spring," exclaimed Liz. "We thought it was from my new guitar, and Zane said he'd had the same kind of thing before, so I ignored it, since it didn't itch or hurt. Besides, it finally went away."

"And Zane is?"

"My boyfriend, the baby's father. So you think I got it from him? What's it going to do to the baby?," Liz asked anxiously. "Zane should have come with me after all."

"Okay, one step at a time," Dr. Garcia said. "First of all, yes, it sounds like you may have contracted syphilis from him. Even if you didn't, he needs to see his doctor to be tested and treated, and you both need to abstain from sex until you are both treated to be sure you don't get reinfected."

"Okay," agreed Liz.

"Secondly, it sounds like you have what we call latent syphilis, meaning that you have no signs or symptoms of syphilis but you still harbor the infection inside you, where it could go on to cause serious damage in the future if it remains untreated. Fortunately, the cure for you is simple—a shot of penicillin today and possibly another penicillin shot later because you are pregnant. The hope is that the penicillin will also completely treat your baby," explained the obstetrician.

"And if it doesn't?," Liz asked fearfully.

"Well, untreated syphilis in pregnancy has up to a forty percent chance of causing miscarriage. Syphilis can also cause blood problems, premature birth, or congenital syphilis in the newborn, meaning the baby can develop multiple problems, including seizures, developmental delays, and problems with its liver, spleen, or nervous system."

"But, as long as we treat this now..."

"We're hopeful that the baby will be fine. We'll be doing blood tests on you throughout your pregnancy to make sure that your treatment is successful, and we'll be able to look closely at your baby with an ultrasound later in the pregnancy to check on him or her," reassured Dr. Garcia.

"Can the penicillin hurt the baby at all?," asked Liz.

"Typically not at this stage of pregnancy. Rarely, the penicillin can trigger a reaction that can lead to miscarriage, but the risk of untreated syphilis is much greater," she explained.

Liz chewed on her lip while she absorbed the information. "So there's no guarantee that my baby will be healthy."

Dr. Garcia placed her hand gently on Liz's arm. "No, Liz, there's not, but there never is. Babies can have defects that no one can predict, but we do screenings like the syphilis test to find and treat everything that we can. That's what prenatal care is all about. Now, unless you have any more questions, I'll send in my nurse with your shot. Please make sure that your boyfriend gets to a doctor and so should any other sexual partners you may have had during the last year or so. If you had the rash last spring, you likely contracted syphilis a couple of months before that."

"Got it," murmured Liz, tears starting to spill down her cheeks. "I know it sounds stupid, but it never occurred to me that there could be something wrong with the baby. I mean, we didn't plan for this pregnancy, but we figured we could handle it. But now, if there're serious problems... Could I please hear the heartbeat before you leave?"

Dr. Garcia reached for the Doppler, and after squeezing jelly on Liz's lower abdomen, quickly picked up the high-pitched, rhythmic whooshing of the baby's heart. "Welcome to parenting, Liz. It's never what you expect."

facts

Syphilis Fact Sheet

What is it?

- Syphilis is caused by a bacterium called Treponema pallidum.

How common is it?

- Syphilis is the least common sexually transmitted infection in the United States, but the numbers are rising. During 2013, there were 17,535 reported cases of primary and secondary syphilis and 56,471 total cases (including primary, secondary, latent, and tertiary syphilis). This is a 10.9% increase in total cases from 2012.

- The year 1990 had the peak number of total cases of syphilis in the United States over the last 50 years: 135,590 cases.

- African Americans have the highest rates (16.8 cases per 100,000 people) compared with Hispanics (6.3 cases per 100,000) and Caucasians (3.0 cases per 100,000) in the CDC's 2013 statistics.

- Men contract syphilis at a much higher rate than women (greater than 10:1), and men who have sex with men (MSM) accounted for 75% of the primary and secondary syphilis cases in 2013.

- Syphilis is often linked with HIV disease.

- Congenital cases are less common, but there are still between 300 and 400 infants born infected with syphilis in the United States each year.

How do you get it?

- Syphilis is transmitted through sexual contact—oral, anal, or vaginal—with an infected person.

- Syphilis can be passed from a mother to her unborn child, causing congenital syphilis.

Where on your body do you get it?

- There are four distinct stages of syphilis:

- The first, or primary, syphilis infection shows up as a small, firm, painless round ulcer, called a chancre, at the site where the bacterium entered the body. These ulcers are usually located on the penis, labia, or vagina, but can also occur on the cervix, in the anus, or in the mouth.

- Secondary syphilis typically presents as a non-itchy skin rash, often on the palms or soles of the feet but sometimes covering more of the body.

- Latent syphilis is untreated syphilis without obvious symptoms.

- Tertiary syphilis can show up anywhere in the body, causing a variety of symptoms, including deafness, blindness, mental illness, heart disease, neurological disorders, and death.

How do I know if I have it?

- Many people are unaware of the initial ulcer because it is painless and can be in a location that can't be easily seen. The ulcer will go away with or without treatment, but the infection remains and may progress.

- If you have a genital ulcer, especially one followed by a rash, a medical professional should examine you and check for syphilis.

- Blood tests can reveal the presence of infection; the blood tests RPR (rapid plasma reagin), VDRL (Venereal Disease Research Laboratory), and FTA-ABS (fluorescent treponemal antibody absorption) all check for antibodies to syphilis.

- A swab of an ulcer can reveal syphilis when viewed under a dark field in the microscope.

What does it look like?

- Primary syphilis is usually a single small, firm, round ulcer on the vagina, labia, penis, or (less often) the mouth or other body location.

- Secondary syphilis looks like red spots on the palms or soles.

- Tertiary syphilis is called the "great imitator" because it can look like such a variety of diseases, depending on which system it affects.

What does it feel like?

- The ulcers of syphilis are typically painless.

- The rash is often not itchy.

- In secondary syphilis, there can be nonspecific symptoms, such as mild sore throat, fatigue, headache, and swollen lymph nodes.

How long does it last?

- Primary syphilis usually breaks out about 3 weeks after exposure but can appear from 9 to 30 days after exposure.

- The chancre will last 3–6 weeks and then will disappear with or without treatment. The infection will persist even when the ulcer leaves, unless antibiotics are used.

- The rash of secondary syphilis occurs 2–10 weeks after the chancre appears, often after the chancre is completely gone. The rash will disappear without treatment but often recurs. Again, the infection will persist unless antibiotics are given.

Can it be cured?

- Yes.

What is the treatment?

- Penicillin is still the treatment of choice for syphilis.

- For people allergic to penicillin, there are alternative antibiotics.

How about alternative therapies?

- No herbs or over-the-counter treatments are effective for syphilis.

Are there long-term consequences?

- Untreated syphilis can lead to neurosyphilis and other forms of tertiary syphilis.

- Tertiary syphilis can cause deafness, blindness, mental illness, heart disease, and death.

When are you contagious?

- Once infected, you are contagious until you are cured with antibiotics. Latent syphilis is the least contagious; primary, secondary, and early latent syphilis are the most contagious.

Can syphilis be transmitted between homosexual partners?

- According to 2013 CDC data, 75% of all new cases of primary and secondary syphilis in the United States occurred in homosexual men.

- There is a case report of woman-to-woman transmission, but this is not thought to be common.

How do I avoid getting syphilis?

- Abstinence from oral, anal, and vaginal intercourse will prevent the transmission of primary syphilis.

- Condoms reduce (but do not eliminate) transmission of syphilis only when they cover an active sore. However, lesions are frequently outside the area sheathed by a condom.

- Secondary syphilis can be contracted through skin-to-skin contact with an infected person; be especially cautious of rashes on people's palms or soles.

If I have syphilis, how do I avoid giving it to my partner?

- Abstain from oral, anal, and vaginal intercourse until both you and your partner have been fully treated for syphilis with appropriate antibiotics.

Frequently Asked Questions

➤ **Can you catch syphilis from a toilet seat?**

No. The bacterium dies when it gets dry.

➤ **Since syphilis has been around for centuries, is it resistant to most antibiotics?**
No. Syphilis still responds to penicillin and other antibiotics.

➤ **Can you have syphilis and not know it?**
Yes, particularly since the initial sores are not painful and often not easily visible.

➤ **When are people tested for syphilis?**
Many states require a blood test for syphilis to obtain a marriage license, and pregnant women are tested to prevent congenital syphilis in their babies.

Additional Information

American Sexual Health Association
PO Box 13827
Research Triangle Park, NC 27709
919-361-8400
www.ashasexualhealth.org/

Centers for Disease Control and Prevention
1600 Clifton Road
Atlanta, GA 30329-4027
1-800-CDC-INFO (1-800-232-4636), 1-888-232-6348 (TTY)
www.cdc.gov/std/syphilis/default.htm

MedlinePlus
US National Library of Medicine
8600 Rockville Pike
Bethesda, MD 20894
1-888-FIND-NLM (1-888-346-3656) or 301-594-5983
www.nlm.nih.gov/medlineplus/syphilis.html

21: Grace's Epilogue

Grace was exhausted. It had been three nights since she had been able to get any decent sleep. On Tuesday night, she had been up tending to her younger daughter, Ann, who had a stomach virus. On Wednesday night, Grace had been on call for her family practice group of six physicians, and with flu season in full gear, her phone seemed to go off every fifteen minutes all night long. Last night, all she had wanted to do was get to bed early, but her husband, Travis, had been on call at the hospital for his cardiology group. This left Grace parenting the kids by herself on a night filled with soccer practice, makeup homework, and a science fair project. Grace had finally made it to bed around eleven thirty, which gave her only six hours to get caught up on sleep before Friday's routine began.

The morning schedule had been packed with the usual mix of patients: people with diabetes, high blood pressure, or depression, as well as everyone with a cough who wanted to be fixed for their weekend activities. Grace looked at the remaining two patients on her schedule. The first was a teenager with a skin problem, and the second was a new patient with a sore throat. "Good," she thought.

"They should both be quick." She glanced down at her watch and was dismayed that it was already two thirty. That would leave her less than forty-five minutes to see these last patients, complete all her charts from the day, and review lab results before she needed to leave to pick up her kids from school.

Grace rarely drank caffeine, but she was craving a pick-me-up to help her through the last hour. She ducked into the break room and grabbed a soda from the fridge. Since the next patient wasn't ready yet, Grace sat down and started typing her notes into the computer records as she drank her soda. Suddenly, Grace realized that she had been ignoring a growing tingling sensation on the right side of her crotch. "Oh man, not today," she thought as her heart sank. But really, it was no surprise after the week she'd had. Grace now had over fifteen years of personal experience dealing with genital herpes, so she had no doubt what it meant when she started feeling burning and tingling on that side of her groin.

It seemed a lifetime ago that she had been a first-year medical student diagnosed with herpes. The first two years had been completely awful. Between lack of sleep, crummy nutrition, and tons of stress, Grace constantly had outbreaks, even after she started taking daily preventive medicines. In fairness, with her on-call schedule, working thirty-six-hour shifts, and losing track of time and days, she had not been able to take the medicines as consistently as she should have. She had to be sure to wear loose cotton underwear, and she had avoided wearing jeans throughout the rest of med school. During her residency, the outbreaks had decreased to every three or four months.

Grace had dated several different men during medical school but had chosen not to be intimate with anyone again until she fell head over heels in love with Travis. She remembered her relief when she had the painful discussion with Travis about her infection and found out that he, too, had a history of genital herpes, which he got when he was in college. Luckily for him, he had only a couple of outbreaks the year he caught it and never had another problem with it. She and Travis had been married for over a decade.

Grace thought about the C-sections she had to have when her children were born because of having an outbreak when she went into labor with her first child. This STI had impacted her life for a long time. She picked up her purse and fished through it until she found her prescription medications. Grace still carried the pills in her purse from force of habit but had rarely needed them for several years. She was happy that it had been almost a year since her last outbreak. She swallowed the pill along with the last of her soda just as her nurse, Vicki, walked around the corner.

"Your next patient is ready," Vicki announced. Then in a quieter voice, she added, "This one might take a bit longer than we originally thought."

Grace stood and took the chart from her nurse. "Isn't this the teenager with acne? Is it that bad?," she asked.

"Not acne. Her skin problem is on her bottom," said the nurse. "By the way, her mom is with her."

Grace exchanged a look of resignation with Vicki and headed down the hallway toward the patient.

"Hi, Meg. Hi, Mrs. Schmid. So, how have you been doing?," Grace asked.

Meg was a volleyball star at a nearby high school. Grace had taken care of her since her early grade-school years but had probably seen her only twice per year on average—once each year for her annual sports-participation physical and sometimes again for an injury or a minor illness. Grace was trying to remember if Meg had mentioned having a boyfriend during her physical last summer.

"I'm doing great, except for this skin thing," replied Meg.

"She has what looks like a spider bite or something," her mom added. "I gave her some antibiotic cream to put on it earlier in the week, but it doesn't look any better to me. I think she's making it worse by scratching it."

"I'm not scratching it, Mom. It doesn't itch, but it kind of stings," said Meg.

"All right. Meg, when did you first notice it?," asked Grace.

"I think it first started last weekend as a little red bump," said Meg.

"But when you showed me on Tuesday, it looked more like several bites," interjected her mother, "and now it's kind of crusted, like it's infected."

"Well, the last time I had one, it looked just like this, and it went away on its own," Meg replied defensively.

"You've had this before?," Grace and Mrs. Schmid said, almost at the same time.

"Yeah. I had a bite like this last semester, but it was higher up, so it didn't rub on my underwear as much. I guess that's why it wasn't as bad," said Meg.

"Have you had these bumps anywhere else on your body?," asked the doctor.

"No, just on the right side of my booty," said Meg.

"Okay. Well, with skin things, a picture is worth a thousand words, so let's take a look, okay?," asked Grace.

"Sure," said Meg, reaching down to pull the gown away.

Grace interrupted her. "Just a minute. Meg, would you like your mom to stay, or would you prefer more privacy?" Grace looked toward Mrs. Schmid. "No offense, of course—but I always like to offer that to teenagers." She was trying to keep her voice light but wanted to communicate to Meg that she might be bringing up issues that could be uncomfortable to discuss with her mother present. Meg's mom understood what was going on immediately, although Meg clearly did not.

"Meg, would you like me to leave? Is there anything you need to discuss in private with the doctor?," she asked intently, leaning forward and looking her daughter straight in the eyes.

Meg shrugged her shoulders and with a quick roll of her eyes said, "Whatever, Mom. It's no big deal." Then she looked at Grace. "Really, it's just a bug bite, or rash, or whatever."

Grace pulled on a pair of gloves. She walked over to the exam table and asked Meg to lie back. Grace lifted the gown and looked down at Meg's bottom. Sure enough, she saw exactly what she was expecting—a cluster of scabbed-over blisters on a bright red base. She also saw a circular dark area higher up on the same side. "Is this where the last one was?," she asked.

Meg twisted her body so she could look where Grace was pointing. "Yeah, right there where that dark spot is now."

Grace tried to be casual. She swabbed the area with the cotton-tipped applicator from the herpes culture kit as she asked, "So, have you noticed any vaginal discharge or irritation with these?"

Meg blushed. "No."

"Okay, then, go ahead and sit up, and let's talk about this for a minute," said Grace.

Before Grace could say anything else, Mrs. Schmid jumped in. "Meg, have you and Kyle been sleeping together?," she asked in a level voice.

Now Meg was bright red but emphatic. "No. We absolutely have not had sex, Mom."

Grace felt like disappearing. She had no doubt that this was herpes. The only question was how to handle the situation with Meg's mother present. Grace preferred to deal with the underage patient one-on-one and then help the patient find a way to communicate the information to the parent.

Luckily, at this point, Meg's mom stood up, clearly struggling with mixed emotions, but quietly and calmly said, "You know what? I think I would prefer it if the two of you discussed Meg's rash alone, and then I'll come back in and you can explain it to me in a few minutes, okay?"

Meg offered a mild protest but looked relieved when her mother was gone. After the door closed, Grace looked at Meg.

"I swear, we have not had sex yet. What is the deal? What do you think this is?" Meg was rattled.

Grace took a breath. "Well, it certainly looks like herpes." She paused a moment while Meg looked at her in shock, tears filling her eyes.

"But really, we have not had sex," she cried.

"Meg," Grace said calmly, "have you had oral sex?"

Meg had now lost all composure. "Yes, but just a few times. That doesn't count, does it?," she sobbed.

"Unfortunately, it does count for this. If he had herpes in his mouth, which is really common, then you could have caught this from oral sex," Grace explained.

"But it's on my rear end, not my front. Trust me, he didn't go there," Meg insisted.

"The herpes virus comes in through the skin but then goes to the nervous system," explained Grace. "When it comes out, it picks one nerve route to travel on, which is why it stays on one side. Most of the time, it does show up a little closer to the labia or vagina, but often it appears on either the front of the leg or on the buttocks, where you have it."

Meg bit her lip and tried to process what she was hearing. Grace knew only too well what was going on in her brain. Part of Grace wanted to hug her, tell Meg that she herself had gotten this infection the exact same way, and share how she had coped with it. Part of her wanted to maintain her professional distance, and part of her just wanted to finish up so she could go get her kids and escape this painful aspect of her job. In the end, Grace's natural compassion won out, and she told Meg the story of her "best friend, Stephanie," in medical school who had suffered from herpes but had learned to deal with it. She taught Meg all about the disease and its treatment and prevention. Grace talked to Meg at length about birth control and other sexually transmittable diseases, though Meg swore that after this, she would never be intimate with her boyfriend again. Finally, Grace asked what Meg would like Grace to tell her mother.

This brought more tears, but Meg composed herself fairly quickly and said with far more maturity than Grace thought that she would have had at seventeen, "You know, I got myself into this. I should be the one to tell her. Will you stay here while I tell her, so you can answer any questions she has?"

"Of course," Grace answered.

She stepped out of the room and asked the nurse to bring back Meg's mother. As Grace checked her watch, Vicki said, "Don't worry, the last patient really is easy. I already did her rapid strep test, and it was positive. We'll get you out in time to get your kids and you can finish your charting tomorrow."

"Thanks, Vicki, you're the best," said Grace with a relieved smile.

She went back into the room, where Meg was already dressed and sitting on the end of the exam table. Mrs. Schmid entered just behind Grace, and they both sat down. Meg didn't wait for any prompting. She looked right at her mom and, with tears still in her eyes, began pouring out her story. "Mom, I didn't lie. We haven't had sex, I promise. But we did get carried away and did, you know, have, um... oral a couple of times last year. Please don't tell Dad, okay?," she ended in a rush.

Her mom looked as though she had been punched but, to her credit, remained calm. She looked at Grace. "We'll talk about your father later. Right now, let's find out what we need to do for you." Mrs. Schmid turned her attention back to Grace and asked, "So, what exactly is her rash?"

"It's herpes," Grace replied.

"And can you give her an antibiotic to make it go away?," asked Mrs. Schmid.

Grace went through most of her explanations about herpes again, concluding by handing Mrs. Schmid a prescription to be filled only if Meg had another outbreak, since it was too late for the antiviral medicine to be helpful for this one. Grace answered a few more questions and then gave them a handout to take home that contained all the information they had gone over. As Grace walked out of the room, she was touched to see Mrs. Schmid get up and silently embrace her daughter in a tight hug. It always impressed her how many parents dealt well with bad news, at least in the office, despite what their children expected.

As a parent herself, Grace knew Mrs. Schmid had to be every bit as upset as Meg, although certainly with a different mix of emotions. The initial anger, fear, and disappointment would give way to the frustration of not being able to protect her daughter from any guy or any disease.

"What am I going to do to help protect my kids from ending up in a situation like this?," she thought. She hoped that raising her children in a medical household would at least make it easier to talk about STIs when they were old enough to understand about sex. They already understood many medical expressions like "respiratory distress" and "cardiac arrhythmia" from listening to their parents' conversations at home. Grace chuckled as she pictured herself shifting the dinner conversation every night of their adolescence, telling story after story of unsuspecting young women and men catching these "gifts that keep on giving."

Sadly, the real stories that her patients shared weekly had so many similarities that they seemed completely predictable to Grace. For example, what happens when a couple ends a long-term relationship, then sleeps together a month or two later for that "one last time" at a point when they are both just feeling lonely? Almost inevitably, one of them walks away from that reunion with a new infection. Or, when does a condom break? Exactly when the woman is ovulating, of course. Would it make a difference if her son and daughters really knew about these patterns and possibilities?

In Grace's experience, it seemed that everyone believed that only society's "undesirables" contracted STIs. In reality, STIs have no bias. However wealthy or well educated, whatever race, gender, or sexual identity, it doesn't matter. If you have sex, you're at risk for getting a sexually transmitted infection. Grace thought about not only her own experience, but also the experiences of her friends. One woman was not able to have children after she got pelvic inflammatory disease from chlamydia. A few of her friends had dealt with genital warts, and Nancy, her childhood neighbor and best friend, had paid the ultimate price, dying from cervical cancer when she was only in her thirties.

In contrast, at this point in her life, Grace recognized that her own genital herpes was merely a hassle, not a serious medical issue. Of course, Grace was aware that this was her mature perspective both as a patient and as a doctor. If only she could bottle this knowledge and prescribe it to Meg, then that would be the next best thing to a cure. Meanwhile, a few pills, a bunch of compassion, and a lot of education would have to do. Grace gave herself a mental fist bump and charged down the hall to see her last patient.

Bibliography

Bailey, J. V., C. Farquhar, C. Owen, and P. Mangtani. "STIs in Women Who Have Sex with Women." *Sexually Transmitted Infections* 80, no. 3 (2004).

Bauer, G. R., and S. Welles. "Beyond Assumptions of Negligible Risk: STDs and Women Who Have Sex with Women." *American Journal of Public Health* 91, no. 8 (2001).

Beauman, John. "Genital Herpes: A Review." *American Family Physician* 72, no. 8 (2005).

Brown, D., and J. Frank. "Diagnosis and Management of Syphilis." *American Family Physician* 68, no. 2 (2003).

Campos-Outcalt, D., and S. Hurwitz. "Female-to-Female Transmission of Syphilis: A Case Report." *Sexually Transmitted Diseases* 29, no. 2 (2002).

Carey, Kate B., Sarah E. Durney, Robyn L. Shepardson, and Michael P. Carey. "Incapacitated and Forcible Rape of College Women: Prevalence across the First Year." *Journal of Adolescent Health* 56, no. 6 (2015).

Centers for Disease Control and Prevention. *HIV/AIDS Surveillance Report, 2006.* Vol. 18. Atlanta, GA: US Department of Health and Human Services, CDC, 2008. www.cdc.gov/hiv/topics/surveillance/resources/reports/.

———. "Sexually Transmitted Diseases Treatment Guidelines." *Morbidity and Mortality Weekly Report* 55 (2006).

———. "Updated Recommended Treatment Regimens for Gonococcal Infections and Associated Conditions—United States." *Morbidity and Mortality Weekly Report* 56 (2007).

Cram, L., M. Zapata, E. Toy, and B. Baker. "Genitourinary Infections and Their Association with Preterm Labor." *American Family Physician* 65, no. 2 (2002).

Fethers, K., C. Marks, A. Mindel, and C. Estcourt. "STIs and Risk Behaviours in Women Who Have Sex with Women." *Sexually Transmitted Infections* 76, no. 5 (2000).

Flinders, D., and P. De Schweinitz. "Pediculosis and Scabies." *American Family Physician* 69, no. 2 (2004).

Grimes, Jill, ed. *Sexually Transmitted Disease: An Encyclopedia of Diseases, Prevention, Treatment, and Issues.* Santa Barbara, CA: ABC-CLIO, 2014.

Jin, F., et al. "Transmission of HSV Types 1 and 2 in a Prospective Cohort of HIV-Negative Gay Men: The Health in Men Study." *Journal of Infectious Diseases* 194, no. 5 (2006).

Khalsa, Ann. "Preventive Counseling, Screening, and Therapy for the Patient with Newly Diagnosed HIV Infection." *American Family Physician* 73, no. 2 (2006).

Kurowski, K. "The Woman with Dysuria." *American Family Physician* 57, no. 9 (1998).

Marr, Lisa. *Sexually Transmitted Diseases: A Physician Tells You What You Need to Know.* 2nd ed. Baltimore, MD: Johns Hopkins University Press, 2007.

Marrazzo, J. M. "Genital HPV Infection in Women Who Have Sex with Women: A Concern for Patients and Providers." *AIDS Patient Care and STDs* 14, no. 8 (2000).

Marrazzo, J. M., K. Stine, and L. Koutsky. "Genital HPV Infection in Women Who Have Sex with Women: A Review." *American Journal of Obstetrics and Gynecology* 183, no. 3 (2000).

McMillan, A., and H. Young. "Rectal Chlamydial Infection among Men Who Have Sex with Men: Partner Notification as a Means of Nucleic Acid Amplification Test Validation." *International Journal of STD and AIDS* 18, no. 3 (2007).

Miller, K. "Diagnosis and Treatment of *Chlamydia trachomatis* Infection." *American Family Physician* 73, no. 8 (2006).

———. "Diagnosis and Treatment of *Neisseria gonorrhoeae* Infections." *American Family Physician* 73, no. 10 (2006).

Moran, J. "Clinical Evidence Concise—Gonorrhea." *American Family Physician* 72, no. 1 (2005).

Moyer, Linda, E. Mast, and M. Alter. "Hepatitis C: Part I. Routine Serologic Testing and Diagnosis." *American Family Physician* 59, no. 1 (1999).

———. "Hepatitis C: Part II. Prevention Counseling and Medical Evaluation." *American Family Physician* 59, no. 2 (1999).

Mravcak, S. "Primary Care for Lesbians and Bisexual Women." *American Family Physician* 74, no. 2 (2006).

Owen, M., and T. Clenney. "Management of Vaginitis." *American Family Physician* 70, no. 11 (2004).

Ribes, J., A. Steele, J. Seabolt, and D. Baker. "Six-Year Study of the Incidence of Herpes in Genital and Nongenital Cultures in a Central Kentucky Medical Center Patient Population." *Journal of Clinical Microbiology* 39, no. 9 (2001).

Roberts, C. M., J. R. Pfister, and S. J. Spear. "Increasing Proportion of Herpes Simplex Virus Type 1 as a Cause of Genital Herpes Infection in College Students." *Sexually Transmitted Diseases* 30, no. 10 (2003).

Shapley, M., J. Jordan, and P. Croft. "A Systematic Review of Postcoital Bleeding and Risk of Cervical Cancer." *British Journal of General Practice* 56 (June 2006).

Smith, Liz. "ACOG Releases Guidelines for Managing Abnormal Cervical Cytology and Histology in Adolescents." *American Family Physician* 74, no. 8 (2006).

Temte, Jonathon. "HPV Vaccine: A Cornerstone of Female Health." *American Family Physician* 75, no. 1 (2007).

US Preventive Services Task Force. "Screening for Chlamydial

Infection: Recommendations and Rationale." *American Family Physician* 65, no. 4 (2002).

Walsh, D. E., R. Griffith, and A. Behforooz. "Subjective Response to Lysine in the Therapy of Herpes Simplex." *Journal of Antimicrobial Chemotherapy* 12, no. 5 (1983).

Warner, L., et al. "Condom Effectiveness for Reducing Transmission of Gonorrhea and Chlamydia: The Importance of Assessing Partner Infection Status." *American Journal of Epidemiology* 159, no. 3 (2004).

Warren, Terri. *The Good News about the Bad News: Herpes: Everything You Need to Know.* Oakland, CA: New Harbinger, 2009.

Westrom, L., and P.-A. Mardh. "Acute Pelvic Inflammatory Disease (PID)." In *Sexually Transmitted Diseases*, 2nd ed., edited by K. K. Holmes, P.-A. Mardh, P. F. Sparling, and P. J. Wiesner, 593–613. New York: McGraw-Hill, 1990.

Index

Library of Congress Cataloging-in-Publication Data

Grimes, Jill.

Seductive delusions : how everyday people catch STIs / Jill Grimes, MD. — second edition

pages cm

Includes bibliographical references and index.

ISBN 978-1-4214-1924-4 (pbk. : alk. paper) — ISBN 1-4214-1924-6 (pbk. : alk. paper) — ISBN 978-1-4214-1925-1 (electronic) — ISBN 1-4214-1925-4 (electronic) 1. Sexually transmitted diseases—Popular works. 2. Self-care, Health—Popular works. I. Title.

RC200.G74 2016

616.95'1—dc23 2015022722